UNITY LIBRARY & ARCHIVES
A study of pleasure and pain.
BJ 1409 .W6

A Study of PLEASURE and PAIN

By ERNEST WOOD

The Theosophical Press
Wheaton, Illinois
1962

CONTENTS

			Page
Chapter	1.	The Value of Pain	1
Chapter	2.	Pain Among the Animals	7
Chapter	3.	Plants, Animals and Babies	13
Chapter	4.	Old Age and the Stages of Life	19
Chapter	5.	Emotional Pain	28
Chapter	6.	The Value of Emotional Pains	40
Chapter	7.	The Cure of Emotional Pains	47
Chapter	8.	The Egoic Pains	55
Chapter	9.	The Pains of Love	67
Chapter	10.	Beyond the Stoics	73
Chapter	11.	Knowledge, Law and Life	86

Books by the same Author

A "Secret Doctrine" Digest

The Seven Rays

The Intuition of the Will

Concentration

Practical Yoga, Ancient and Modern

The Glorious Presence

Great Yoga Systems

Mind and Memory Training

Yoga Dictionary

Yoga (Penguin Series)

Zen Dictionary

CHAPTER 1

The Value of Pain

"Rejoice, O my heart, for we are alive!"

Every moment since these words were written, millions of people have been silently uttering them. It is, as it were, the anthem of conscious existence. "It is good to be alive." "Of all the things for which we are thankful, we are thankful for the gift of life."

"Yes, yes," says the modern, thinking man, "but there is an if." If only it could be free from pain—the pains of the body (so many accidents and infirmities), and the pains of the mind, (so many insecurities, frustrations and indignities). "How grand it would be if only there were no pain." Many people have, no doubt, thought of life in heaven as life without pain.

Let us see, however, what this pain is and what it does. We are modern people, who have found a good use for nearly everything in this world; can we see the nature and utility of pain in living organisms?

In ourselves we find a variety of pains. There are at least five kinds of it—(1) physical or bodily pain, as in the case of various hurts and injuries and in certain kinds of diseases; (2) emotional pain, such as we experience when we cannot get or we lose some object we very much want; (3) mental pain when we are unable to understand the conditions in which we find ourselves or when we find some weakness in a cherished belief or idea; (4) social pain, when we are parted from our beloved relatives and friends, or are plagued by incompatible workmates, neighbors and enemies, and (5) egoic and moral pains when we are discontented with our status or have occasion to reproach ourselves for our shortcomings.

I wish to review in the first place the general course of development of these several pains, and how they are related to their respective pleasures. First, let us notice that low grades of beings are very inert or sluggish, and that it takes a certain kind of pain to stir them into activity—I refer to hunger. An old scripture of India says: "Life is hunger, hunger is life." This goes behind our stock modern scientific statements that living creatures are characterized by having an instinct of self-preservation. The babe that cries is not thinking about self-preservation, he is not like the wild animal that sleeps with "one eye open or one ear cocked." He is hungry. He is merely hungry, and to that extent in pain. When the babe finds the breast and begins to suck the milk, he is visibly not merely relieved from pain but positively enjoying pleasure. So the relief of the hunger is not merely a reverse effect, removing the pain of the hunger, but is geared to a new experience, namely, pleasure.

All this is very undefined in the very early days, but gradually there arises the seeking of pleasure without the goad of hunger. In this stage there is the recognition that there are various pains associated with certain things and various pleasures associated with certain other things. From this desires arise—desires to avoid and desires to obtain. These desires when remembered or thought of in the mind are emotions—they cause motion outward, action in reference to things. Certain things are pain-causing, so they are disliked and avoided; other things are pleasurable, so they are liked and are sought. Sometimes, when action is blocked by conditions and circumstances, the emotions are pent-up, and then they have a peculiar pain of their own.

In the early stages it is not realized that the pleasures become painful if there is too much of them. It is at this stage that we can best see the importance of naturalness in these matters. The child has arisen from a father and a mother who have bodies made up of certain functions and structures. These bodies have gradually become as they are because of their living in a certain kind of environment. Thus we human beings have a set of sense-organs (ears, eyes, nose, etc.) and a set of action-organs (hands, feet, mouth, etc.) and these are maintained in a body which breathes and requires a certain amount of air, which digests and requires a certain amount of food. With regard to this food (to follow up our example) the pursuit of pleasure to the extent of taking in an excess quantity will result in pain in the body, because there is a violation of the order of nature, long-established through many generations.

So the pursuit of pleasure to this extent brings about another set of pains. This results in the development of the intellect. "Why did that third helping of apple pie give me stomach ache?" "Because you took too much!" There are dozens of violations of bodily naturalness, or health, which bring about disease (dis-ease) and pains, and the human being had better use his intelligence with regard to all these. This intelligence was not only promoted by bodily pain in the first place, but also because of his wrong or unnatural use of external things. And even the things of the body are concerned not merely with proper eating, but also proper exercise, proper rest and proper protection by houses and clothing.

Considering all these things, we see that not only is this intellect stirred up in the first place by pains resulting from wrong desires and goaded on to further efforts by more pains and new pains resulting from its own errors, but it also grows when and while it is being used. It comes to the point where it makes plans and designs for new things in its life, to reduce pains and increase pleasures. Then comes the pleasure of knowing and the pleasure of thinking. This is a big field of enhancement of life—the sense of living, and the joy of life—so that as adult human beings we find ourselves compositely living with three hungers—hunger for physical, emotional and mental satisfactions and pleasures.

Looking back for a moment we see that at every stage it was pain that promoted the activity and enhancement of life—physically, hunger; emotionally, the avoidance of things disliked; mentally, the solving of problems, and the struggle for the enlargement of living. Away in the far past we picture the cave man and primitive man. Comparing that man with present man we see that what he has and what he is are vastly greater than what he had and what he was. We see also that every bit of that greatness was won by his own efforts in dealing with the things around him and to some extent with himself. In one of the old Hindu books there is a curiously paradoxical statement about man. It describes him as "the powerful, and powerless, the ignorant, the wise." And that is what we actually find. Man is born the most helpless creature in the world, without natural clothing or weapons, without swiftness or acute senses, without the instinct to build a house or take the food that suits his needs.

We might think, if we were not evolutionists, that if God created this world he had some curious reason for discriminating against man, to form him thus helpless and unprotected against the creatures of the world. But what do we find in effect? That physical disadvantage and difficulty and mental growth have gone on together. Man without natural clothing can live in every climate of the world, because with the aid of his mind he provides it for himself, suited to the places where he wants to go or live. Man, without natural strength or weapons, has made for himself innumerable tools and machines and engines with which he has made himself partner in the forces of Nature, and wielder of the weapons of thunder and lightning, conqueror of every other creature by virtue of the mind with its ever-increasing knowledge and understanding, and its moral instinct to associate with other men. Man, without wings, can soar higher and further and faster than any bird and he can travel across oceans and continents in a few hours. With the instruments of science he can see the distant and the small, talk to his neighbor three thousand miles away, and send his messages in a moment round the world on the wings of invisible ether. He can record his thoughts for his neighbor and the use of future generations. He can understand and enjoy beauty and humor, and produce instruments of entrancing melody and harmony and glorious works of art. And amid all these achievements a still greater thing has come to him—a rich inner life of the mind, the result of his experiences and efforts, every day growing fuller and more able to cope with the still larger and more far-reaching experiences and teachings of this marvellous world of life. In the midst of this, how can it be said that the difficulties and troubles of life have not proved of benefit to man, helping to give him the one thing that all thoughtful men value above everything else—a rich and powerful consciousness? In these circumstances we can cease objecting to pain as such, and begin to accept the idea that the world is the friend of man.

If we may allow ourselves a look at the fictional or allegorical story of Adam and Eve in the Garden of Eden and afterwards, we may find something of the same lesson that trouble and pain have a prime value. Those two people were having a life of ease and simple pleasure, with no ambition or intellectual interests to set them to work, and no doubt they had a certain degree or quality of conscious life which might have gone on for an indefinite time in just the same way, but for the intervention of something that disturbed that placid continuum. There was some movement of curiosity, of unfulfilled desire, in Eve, which caused her to grasp the fruit of a tree which when eaten would enable her to know good and evil—perhaps the good and the bad would be a clearer statement, for the idea seems to be that they began to see the varying values of things around them as ministering to their pleasure, which could hardly have been all at one dead level of interest and satisfaction. In taking this fruit Adam and Eve disobeyed the injunction or impulse to be contented with things as they turned up, without examining them and selecting among them. The devil was perhaps this arising mental curiosity, which certainly does seem to have been going on its belly ever since, rather than reaching to higher and happier things. Be that as it may, the fact was that those two people now found themselves in the outer world, where they had to earn their living by the sweat of the brow. Why of the brow? It seems to imply thought as well as action. It was not simply because of disobedience that they were turned out of Eden; on the contrary, the account clearly states that it was because they might have proceeded further and eaten the fruit of another tree, the tree of life. We must call it, I think, the tree of immortal life, because they already had life, and eating the fruit of it would have made them able to live forever—not mere human beings which presumably they were, even in Eden. Now, very interestingly this second tree comes up again at the other end of the Bible, in The Revelation of St. John. It there states as a message from Jesus Christ that to him who overcometh shall be given to eat the fruit of the tree of life, which stands in the midst of the paradise of God. St. Paul also was very much concerned with overcoming this mortal state of ours, which he regarded as a more or less semi-dead state—so much so that he could declare to certain of his followers: "Ye are dead, and your life is hid with Christ in God." But Jesus himself had sown the seed for these ideas about overcoming and immortal life, when he said: "I have overcome the world."

What I am trying to say is that it was not a bad thing that those people were turned out of Eden and had to face pain and perform labor of body and mind, for without that they could presumably never have enjoyed the fruit of that second tree. And the business of overcoming looks very much like a sort of evolution through self-effort, followed by sudden acquisition of realization of immortal life, when they had learned to understand and master this world of semi-death—or world of obstruction—with all its human problems. Briefly, all this pain was not a bad thing, but was a challenge to these people to go in and win right to the very top; such that again Paul could describe it in one of his numerous exhortations, as "unto the measure of the stature of the fulness of Christ." And here it seems "stature of the fulness" is significant, being redolent of achievement, while "fulness of the stature" might have contained a touch of the idea of acquisition and accumulation rather than the sudden translation to immortality which was promised.

I have cited this case to show that religion is not at war with science in seeing the great value of pain and trouble.

We have now to consider pain among the animals and also the question whether this value of pain has reference to the individual human being, and not merely to the race of man, as we have shown.

Chapter 2

Pain Among the Animals

Without attempting to define or formulate the nature of life, I wish to state that animals are living beings, and there is pain in their lives. Just as is the case with man, these creatures are responding with pain and with pleasure to the various contacts of outside objects and conditions—also to the results of their own actions which make contact with various things in various ways.

Bodily pain and bodily pleasure occur at the point where life meets forms. Our life is sometimes defined in terms of that meeting. Ask the average man what his life is, and quite probably he will say, "Oh, I get up in the morning, take a shower, come downstairs and have breakfast, drive to the job, lay the bricks, take lunch and perhaps talk a bit, lay some more bricks, drive back home, eat again, take the wife out or play with the children, and then go back to bed." It is a series of contacts which take place on a line of time.

At the points of contact the man may be active in all three ways—physically, emotionally and mentally—or, quite often in only two ways and, even more rarely, in only one. Examples of the "only one" type are men in almost explosive outbursts of activity, men in tearing rages or in panic, and men in deep thought. In such cases the consciousness of self for the time being is as of only an acting being, only an emotional self or only a mental self. It happens also that, in most people, the self when "in repose" is liable to relapse mainly into one of these, rather than to present itself to itself with a balance of the three.

Now, the animals and man have acquired their present bodily forms with their particular kinds of sense organs and action organs, as the result of these contacts and the reactions they engender. So life exists on a line of time, and it is to be observed that the material things on that line of time are resisting change, while the living beings are trying to make changes, on account of the hunger (or pain) which has already been described.

To say that material things resist change (except mechanical or chemical predictable reactions) and that life has hunger or hungers that demand change, leads to the following definitions: Matter is that which carries the past into the present; life (including mind, which is to be discussed later) is that which brings the future into the present. As an example of the latter: If the housewife decides to drive her car tomorrow morning to the market to get some groceries to satisfy the children's hunger and her own, tomorrow morning will see that car going along the road in the required direction. If, however, there is no such or similar decision on the part of the housewife, that car will just stand there in the garage and present us with a repetition of what was there yesterday—or perhaps we should say a continuation of the past into the present.

Life can, however, act on the forms and alter them to some extent. By such action its own form or body also becomes modified. These modifications of the living being involve an intake, a transformation of the intake into an addition to the existing form, and an elimination of what is not useful for that purpose. The living body becomes more elaborate and more efficient. The well-known process of evolution occurs, which was defined by the famous scientist Herbert Spencer, as follows:

"Evolution is a progressive change from a state of incoherent homogeneity to a state of coherent heterogeneity of structure and function."

Homogeneity is simplicity and uniformity of content, as in the case of homogenized milk, and in the earlier and lower forms in nature these homogeneous parts do not act for the maintenance of one another. Heterogeneity is variety, and coherence is the mutual maintenance of these varied parts, as, for example, in the case of the human body, there are eyes, lips, hands, legs and I do not know how many other organs or instruments. It has been said that legs are being used for seeing when they carry our eyes into another room to observe something there, and eyes are used for walking when they look forward to see where the leg may safely put its foot.

Increased variety and coherence are, so to say, the reward of efforts by the life to avoid pain and obtain pleasure. In this connection it is necessary to notice that these two—pain and pleasure—are so related to the efficiency of the body that when it is impaired there is dis-ease and pain, and when its correctness according to its regular state of development in natural evolution is restored there is pleasure. Pleasure and pain, though a pair of opposites psychologically, are not so practically. They are not two extremes, two ends of a stick. In that stick pleasure is in the middle and pain is at both ends. Let the bath-water be at the right temperature for the body, and there is pleasure; let it get much colder or much hotter and there is pain. So much are pleasure and pain geared to naturalness in the body and its present status in evolution. I knew a man who had asthma for some years, and got better from it; he used to say to others, on occasion, "You people do not seem to realize the pleasure of breathing."

I believe all of us who are observers and thinkers, and have paid any attention to what is happening and has happened to living beings in the field of nature are evolutionists, and to some extent Darwinists. We have observed that in the course of life, as generation succeeds generation, beneficial variations tend to be preserved, and unfavorable variations tend to their own non-continuance through incompetence and death.

We have struck here one of the things about which there is the greatest outcry—that is, death. "Why death?"

Our scientific evolutionists ought to be more attentive to this question. The answer to it is simple. Death is universal among the living organic beings in nature because it is so useful, so beneficial; and because it is the greatest promoter of life—more life, better life.

From the scientific standpoint, which the present writer maintains and which he requests the reader seriously to consider, people ought to have realized long ago that periodical death is one of those occurrences in life which have been preserved and built into the organisms for the simple reason that they are good for life. They advance the life, enrich it, enhance it.

The best is preserved, and the inferior dies out, in the course of the struggle for existence in this world. To be brief: "The best lion gets the worst antelope." When a family of antelopes are fleeing from some lions, they do not run in and out between the scrub bushes of the desert. They glide over them with a smooth and seemingly effortless motion which is a wonder and a delight to behold. I speak of this from experience, having watched them, especially in Kathiawar, in India, in my younger days; and I was sure that those motions were not only a delight to me to behold, but they were also a delight to them to enjoy—they constituted for the antelope a large part of their joy of living. We are bound to notice also that the beauty of limb and motion there to be seen also contributes to our enjoyment and advancement of life. My life is richer for that experience, and in my memory the joy of it and the thanks for it will, I believe, never fade.

The best lion, foremost in its group, gets the benefit of the exercise of its limbs and organs, and is also assured of the greatest probability of survival and procreation, while the worst antelope loses survival and procreation, which are ensured to the better antelopes in the special line of their activity and development. Thus future lions and future antelopes both have an improvement and enhancement of life. In this "survival of the fittest" what is beneficial to the continuance and advancement of the form is preserved in the struggle. There is an improvement in the limbs of the antelope and in the skill and speed of the lions in the case we have cited.

Similarly, in the competition, as we may call it, between mind and matter in the process of living they are improved by each other. There is evolution thereby in the life as well as in the form. We can say of this: "It is still more good now than it was before to be alive." "Rejoice, O my heart, for we are alive!"

has added meaning or quality.

Even by merely seeing and understanding this principle of progress in nature, we also have some enhancement of life, in the mental and emotional departments (so to speak) of our consciousness, and to some extent in our ethical department as well, for we have as a result more fellow feeling towards both lions and antelopes than we had before. It may go so far as to be called "some love for them" which we had not before—love, which always seems to be whispering, "Thank you for being there."

I have another instance in mind of the benefit of this working of nature. When I was visiting San Francisco, some forty years ago, I heard the story of the king of the seal rocks lying off the coast. Some years ago there lived there a huge seal which had been leader of the herd for about a hundred and twenty years; but one day it happened that another seal, a powerful fellow, came up from the south, and made battle with the old king. The two fought, it is said, for three days, and the end came when the old seal, wounded in many places, swam across to the shore and died, and the new king reigned in his stead.

This was an example of what the poet called, "Nature, red in tooth and claw," and it sometimes strikes the imagination as a terrible condition of life.

But consider the consciousness rather than the body of the animal, and there are some things there to be seen which make us pause before we decide. That animal had not the power of man's mind with which it could ruminate in old age upon the experiences of life. Its enjoyment lay in the use of its physical powers, and when those were waning perhaps it was an excellent arrangement that its body should be brought to an end in a grand climax of excitement—the culminating period of its life. I sometimes think with regard to the red-in-tooth-and-claw theory that we are too much the slaves of imagination when we view Nature's arrangements with horror. I remember once carefully watching a struggle between a large grasshopper and a small lizard which had grasped it in its mouth. The lizard was trying to gobble the big insect up, and the grasshopper was kicking with all its legs, and it occurred to me that perhaps from the standpoint of consciousness both these primitive creatures were enjoying the greatest sensations of their lives.

We have observed that certain large rhythms have made themselves evident in this business of the production and preservation of better forms. Death is only one of these rhythms, but one of the most useful. For the benefits to accrue to the antelope tribe it is quite necessary for the relatively unfit to die, and preferably without offspring. It is also necessary for the offspring to have new bodies in which the superior qualities somehow handed on are not mere modifications of the old ones, but consist essentially of the good that has been gained. The embryo does not merely run over the history of the race to which it belongs, as is usually supposed. Somewhere in that gestatory process there must be some sort of competition in which the new genes gain an advantage. At any rate, something of the kind is implied in the observations of a very eminent anthropologist and former President of the Royal Anthropological Institute, London, Sir Arthur Keith, who wrote: "There is a recapitulation of ancestral history as the human embryo passes through its ripening stages, but this recapitulation is masked by the display of characters which are wholly of recent origin. Nor need this surprise us. What should we think of a builder who, in the erection of a palace, insisted on 'recapitulating' all the evolutionary stages which lie between a hut and a palace? In the development of the human body, as of that of every other living thing, we find a strict observance of the principle of economy. If an ancient feature is reproduced, it is because it is a necessary part of the scaffolding for the new."[1]

---

[1]*Concerning Man's Origin,* by Prof. Sir Arthur Keith, p. 21.

Chapter 3

Plants, Animals and Babies

There is much more "hit and miss" method in the procreation of plants than in that of animals. A tree drops thousands and thousands of seeds. Of these only a few fall on fertile ground in a favorable environment, but even in this case we can see that there are small variations in seeds, and some of them will be strong enough to survive in places where others cannot. These survivors, we may say, are on the whole the most competent for carrying on and furthering the characteristics in which the tree is competent. It is said, rightly or wrongly, that probably no two leaves on all the oak-trees in the world have ever been exactly the same. If that is so, let us add that no two acorns have ever been exactly the same.

It has been pointed out by students of biology and sociology that of children born and reared in slums and crowded poverty-stricken areas a much smaller percentage survive than in the more favored families. The figures I quoted when I was writing my books on these subjects back in the 1920's, show that in the slums of the very depressed factory workers of Bombay the mortality of babies within the first year of life was about eighty per cent. And yet that population was increasing, because there were still more children than parents among them at the parental average age of about thirty years. In contrast with this I took, as an example, the case of all the married clergymen in New South Wales—a very intelligent and clean-living class—and showed that the incidence of infant mortality among them was very low, and yet in all those families the average number of children was only about one-and-a-half—a decreasing population. I knew very well one family of business people—somewhere between the two I have mentioned in social status, but well-to-do economically—in which I observed that the grandparents on the father's side had seven children—all married and beyond the age of child-bearing at the time of which I am speaking, and all gently nurtured in childhood. There were five boys and two girls. The five boys had respectively 0, 2, 3, 2 and 1 children; the two girls had 2 and 2 children. These 12 grandchildren (from 14 parents) all got married in due course, and all were sufficiently well-to-do and gently nurtured. I could not trace the further history of some of these, but I do know about the set of 3 above-mentioned—they and their wives, the whole six of them had produced only one child, and that one is now unmarried and over age for child-bearing, being a woman.

In the case of the trees mentioned, it is quite possible that if the inferior seeds (from the standpoint of the kind of tree's qualities) could survive as well as the superior seeds, and then multiply, the tribe would not advance in evolution. I am trying to present the case for "survival of the fittest" in the plant kingdom.

In the human case, the survival of the fittest in the struggle for existence has in all civilized nations—that is, almost everywhere—become a thing of the past. There is now what is called sexual selection—miscalled, I think, because when the teen-agers "fall in love" there is really only a childhood interest in some physical qualities of the loved-one; however strong that "love" may be it is the child-interest in the affairs of the developing senses which creates the attraction, and contact and simple sexuality do the rest. I hope to show the nature and action of child-interest a little further on in this book, and also the fact that there is no such thing as sexual *selection,* the function being quite undiscriminatory. How many teen-agers explain that they were carried away by the impulse to mate, quite unintentionally, after what was only a sensuous exploration and enhancement of touch in the form of kissing and "necking." However, of this more anon.

Now we may consider the matter when the people are married, and between the ages—more or less—of twenty and forty years. This wedding also is not sexual selection. It is emotional selection. The emotional urges to expansion—enhancement of emotion—are now more prominent and more urgent than the impulse to enhancement of the senses. Of this, also more anon. The point here is that mere sexuality is not making any selection.

Mankind no longer has the benefit of what we may call Darwinian natural selection for the improvement of his species, because of our social advancement in brotherly love, with its rejection of the old doctrine and practice of "each for himself, and Devil take the hindmost." Mitigating this sad situation—sad as regards our evolution—there is something which we call social selection. Sometimes this is nothing more than the appreciation of the gently nurtured for the gently nurtured, a social and largely an economic comfort and convenience which is composed very largely of the same emotional considerations—or rather reachings—as those already mentioned. But sometimes in this milieu there is a new factor, due to knowledge and education—mental considerations as to the evolutionary benefit of the proposed marriage, the proposed combination.

It seems, does it not, that mankind, or at any rate the superior classes of mankind, simply must sooner or later desist from the old method of marriage on sensuous (I do not say sensual) and emotional grounds, if the race is to progress. It is all nonsense to say that the sensuous and emotional contacts arise and should be respected because the people are "in love." It is only sexuality. Love is quite another matter, and is—I will venture to say here and explain later—something as superior to intellect as intellect is superior to the emotions groupable under the headings of liking and disliking.

It is not suggested here that young adults should request their more experienced parents or elders, or some incorporated body of experts, to select their mates for them, because the use of their own intelligence in this business of selection is obviously part of the process of their development. Men do not advance by being told what to do, but by using their own human faculty of intelligence whenever it is reasonably feasible to do it. Obviously it would not do for a man to walk down Fifth Avenue or the Bois de Boulogne wearing a skirt instead of trousers, even if he did think it a more comfortable and healthy garment, because of its effect on others —yes, even their stupidity must be bowed to, to some extent.

But the proposal to use intelligence before mating is not of that kind. One may listen also to the opinions of respected elders in this matter, and then make one's decision, without flouting either emotions or sensations—it is not suggested that the young man should marry an ugly girl or one emotionally incompatible. This is part of the elimination of the unfit, through the use of intelligence.

The object of our study of plants and animals in these matters is the better to understand man, so that he may attend to his own future betterment, in circumstances and in himself, since natural selection will not do this for him, and sexual selection cannot, for there is no such thing.

We are concerned primarily with evolution and its requirement of increase of variety of structures and functions, or improvement of such as we have, and its increase of "coherence" or co-ordination. In this matter of coherence we have a principle which even the intellect must bow before and serve. It cannot aim at the advancement of one organ or function without reference to its harmony with the others. But it may well be concerned—in connection with mating or otherwise—in strengthening a weak part, or in making an advance in some particular salient of human progress, such as art, literature or science.

This principle of co-ordination or unity is so fundamentally present and powerful that the body—of plant, animal or man—cannot be said to be a mere accumulation of parts, accretions or alliances. This is seen in the fact that the parts derive their character from the whole, not the reverse. Suppose, for example, we came to some place where a lot of fingers were just lying about. We would then see those pieces of flesh, bone, skin, etc. having a certain shape, but (assuming that we had never seen fingers at work on a hand) it would never occur to us that they were fingers. No, a finger is a finger only on the hand, and a hand is a hand only on the arm; indeed, fingers and hands have grown to be what they are because of the power of unity brought forward by the life. This power seems to be essentially the emotion of self—and later—in its further development—an idea of self. Such appears to be the origin of organic living forms, though to the average evolutionist the significance and even the existence of this original power is often obscured by the bare and bald word "coherence."

I have often noticed how the experience of self, the emotion of self, and the idea of self, arise successively in the life of a baby. First, no doubt, it passively receives the comforts which the mother provides, and sleeps between times. Next, it begins to like certain things and dislike other things; perhaps I should have said situations rather than things, for it has not yet distinguished things as such, nor associated particular forms with its liking and disliking. The mother is at this stage only a comfortable cloud, so to say—but even the word cloud is much too precise. Later it begins to distinguish particular things, and starts to identify them and to associate them with its feelings of liking and disliking. Then, when—and only when—it has discovered things *as things* with precise boundaries and characteristics (in certain respects), it discovers its own identity as one of the things among the many things that are all around.

This process of entification is one that we see also slowly emerging in the large field of Nature. We can say, I think, that in the plants there is some sort of rudimentary feeling, such as for the sunshine and the rain. It is no longer a purely passive thing. Would it be too speculative to suggest that there might be a passive enjoyment of some kind even in the mineral, associated perhaps with its resistivity and elasticity? Anyhow in the plant we can be more confident, especially if we have read about the work of J. C. Bose and others in this connection.

There is, next, quite a radical distinction between a plant and an animal. The plant is rooted to one spot, but reaches out from its root. The animal goes about and contacts a considerable variety of things. (Man, to run ahead for a moment, goes further still and creates new forms for his own use and entertainment.) The meeting of the animal with many things, and the responses by it to this variety, no doubt result in its development of that elementary mental operation which we speak of as "recognition." We need not assume that the animal *thinks* about the objects, nor even remembers them in their absence. But it does recognize them. Knowledge arises when this is there—knowledge which is something more than seeing, for the animal knows from previous experience that water cannot be walked over, and that trees cannot be walked through but must be walked round. Such recognitions—not memories—can be stored in quantity in the elementary mind of the animal, and no doubt constitute the basis of its instincts. One may observe here incidentally, that the plants, in their reachings out and their feelings about, may well be laying the foundations of an elementary emotional nature. This, on the principle that function precedes structure, as seen in the amoeba.

It is worth noticing that in ourselves we have something that corresponds to the distinction between recognition and memory. It may happen, for example, that we have met a Mrs. Pemberton-Jones at a party, and someone speaks about her next day, and says, perhaps, "You remember her, don't you? She was the woman with the big nose." Still we do not remember her, but as chance will have it she just then calls in on her round of visits with a friend. Immediately, you exclaim, "Ah, now I remember." You don't remember; you only recognize. Without a new encounter you would probably never have remembered her.

I take it, then, that the animal mind usually goes so far and no further, and that it is the privilege of man to conjure up pictures of the past on the screen of his memory, and juggle them into new patterns in his present thinking, perhaps with a view to putting those new patterns into action and effect in the world in the near or far future.

Chapter 4

Old Age and the Stages of Life

There is, in that beautiful poem of Sir Edwin Arnold's, *The Light of Asia*—a book which gives us Western people an account of the life and teachings of Buddha—a passage which strikes the reader with something of a shock, and has caused many people to regard Buddhism as presenting an especially gloomy assessment of our human life. Addressing the public in general, it says:

> Ache of the Birth, ache of the helpless days,
>   Ache of hot youth and ache of manhood's prime;
> Ache of the chill grey years and choking death,
>   These fill your piteous time.

A perusal of the Christian Gospels also reveals a considerable preoccupation with the subject of pain, but—strangely enough—it is not so much actual pain that is mentioned as the pains of resentment and frustration. Jesus came to a definitely unhappy people. They deeply resented their position under the heel of the Romans, although they were not too badly off economically, for those days. They remembered the promise of Jehovah to make them a favored nation, a kingdom of priests, and a treasure to him above all people—which he could do because the whole earth was his and as Moses put it, he was a man of war. This Lord had helped them to conquer the Amorites, the Moabites, the Perizzites, the Canaanites, the Hittites, the Girgashites, the Hivites and the Jebusites, whereby the Lord said, "I have given you a land for which ye did not labor, and cities which ye built not, and ye dwell in them; of the vineyards and olive-yards which ye planted not do ye eat."[2]

Besides, there was the prophecy of the coming Messiah, which also helped to keep their resentment and their hope still strong.

[2] Joshua 24, 13.

So they were preoccupied with their collective or tribal effort to achieve their kingdom to such an extent that the welfare of the individual among them was conspicuously subordinated to the communal ambition, and it was only with the coming of the prophets some hundreds of years later that the individual's welfare began to receive its due consideration, and to be regarded also as a subject of the Lord's solicitude. Jesus carried this message of the prophets to its high point, converting the Lord at last into a father caring for his children individually and dealing with them individually, sending his messenger to declare this relationship and stating that the kingdom to be established was "not of this world." Yet still it was a kingdom, and high places were to be competed for in the court of heaven. Certainly the coming leader was to relieve all this pain, even though it was mostly emotional.

Buddha, on the other hand, though born to the purple, was surrounded by simple agrarian people with no ambition but that of carrying on their peaceful human labors and bringing up families as their ancestors had done for a very long time and as their descendants were also expected to do. There was no glory on earth in view in their religion, and so a life well spent, or a series of lives well spent, was anticipated to result in nirvana, not a kingdom in the heavens, but rather, if we must define it from the human limited point of view, a delightful condition of everlasting rest, yet in some sense of joyful life at the same time. It was not thought of as a kingdom, at all events. And what at first stirred Buddha into his search for the truth about human life and the destiny of man was not even the thought that people might look forward to enjoying conspicuous pleasures, but the feeling that surely there must be a means of relief from their multitude of pains and troubles. After considerable study of what the thinking men in his country already knew, and after a great deal of meditation, he realized the "truth" that the pains of life we have listed in this chapter were all due to ignorant desire for the things that perish. The list ends with the pains of old age and death. "The chill grey years" sounds very miserable.

I submit, however, that although Buddha pictured the attainment of nirvana as the final goal of every human life, he also held that the stages of life, including old age, were troubled with pain only when a person was guilty of foolish desires and actions based upon them. I hope to show in these pages that old age can be the most fruitful period in our lives. To this end I must first give an account of the theory of the succession of periods—not Shakespeare's gloomy list, but a set of four, described in old Hindu books as childhood (the learning and developing period), then the family-and-business period, thirdly the thoughtful or studious period, and fourthly the meditative or synthesizing period. These are definitely periods in which the physical, emotional, mental and, shall we say, ethical-spiritual impulses and developments predominate.

Before we go into these in some detail, let me refer to the culmination, old age, as something which has been retained in the course of evolution because it is useful—useful to the individual particularly concerned and also in the field of social development.

Old age, too, or at least aging, must have been built into the organism and preserved in it as a beneficial process. We do not find very much of this in the lower organisms—as explained in our story of the seal—but when we come up to man, the organic being who has by far the most mind, we see the benefits of old age and also how they are transmitted.

My Hindu friends of earlier days used to set great store by this doctrine, much emphasized in their classical literature, regarding the four stages of life. The chief point of it was that all these four stages are beneficial, including old age. All agreed that the first stage was the learning and developing period, the second the family and business period, the third the studious period, and the fourth the meditative or synthesizing period.

Let us, for the sake of clarity, regard these in a modern way as periods of approximately twenty-one years each. In the first —or childhood—period the activity is centered mainly on the development of the senses and the motor organs of the body.

The child is not willing merely to see a "curious object," it wants to feel and handle it as well, and perhaps in the earlier stages to pop the thing into its mouth or lick it. With increasing complexity and subtlety the process goes on through the "teens." I have already mentioned that when the teenager falls in love, as he thinks, it is not really love. He is interested in the long golden hair, or the mysterious dark hair, with its delightful feeling and smell, and its cave-like wonders, and in all those feminine ways of smile and voice and gesture which most mothers are so busy in cultivating in their young daughters.

Thus teen-age love, so-called, is just the same process of sense-interest—nothing more. The loved one can truly be said to be the most liked and most wanted thing in the youth's life, but only for this reason, and in the main it is exploratory. Real love may come about later on, in the second or the further stages —speaking of general or average or normal persons, of course.

It must be emphasized that this first stage of life is very important. I am of the opinion that in families in which there has been repression of the children's childhood impulses involving sense-interest and action-interest, and too much emotional training or mental training, the children have ended up as adults lacking some degree of reality of living and lacking also enterprise, the impulse to action. The reason for this deficiency of development of organs and lack of this awakening, which is almost impossible of recovery in the later stages of life, is that not only the sense-organs are themselves insufficiently developed to respond as closely as should have been the case to the externally contacted objects of the world, but also the inner conscious response which we call life lacks some awakening—in quality and in intensity.

This principle is easy to illustrate. When I was teaching classes for the development of the mind some years ago, I often made use of a device such as the following:

The teacher suddenly brings out some small object of a familiar kind, let us say a pencil, and asks, "What is the color of this?" The students answer, "Yellow." The teacher asks them to close their eyes and think of that yellow color. "Have you got it?" he asks. "Oh, yes," is the answer. "Well, then, open your eyes and look again at this pencil," holding it forward to them. "Look carefully; does it not look yellower than it did before?" In nine cases out of ten the students would say, with some surprise—sometimes with much surprise—"Why, yes, it does!"

The teacher has then succeeded in causing the students to pay closer attention to this act of visual experience than they did before. This has positively improved their visual organs, and it has awakened or enhanced their conscious response. They are now more alert to the world in this respect, and more alive in themselves. It is very useful, I understand, in the teaching of music, to induce the students to obtain a very exact experience of particular notes, before proceeding to their combination in chords or in melodies.

This is what children are doing—developing their organs and awakening themselves—when they lend themselves to curiosity and apparently aimless expressions of their organs of action. This is why they tire so soon of their toys; when according to their individual capacities they have extracted what they can of benefit from those toys. But if the toys are too many, or too rapid in succession, the later toy will distract the attention from the earlier toy too soon. I have often told the story of the little boy in the drug-store, sitting there on a high stool joyously licking his ice-cream cone. Two men were looking on. One said to the other, "You know, that little boy does not like ice-cream." "Oh," came the rather sour reply, "I suppose you are going to say that he only likes the taste of the ice-cream." "No," said the first man, "He does not even like the taste of the ice-cream. All he likes is the consciousness of the taste of the ice-cream."

It is only the consciousness, the life, that we all like, and even so not when it is standing still but only when it is being enhanced.

In the second period of twenty-one years the emotions have primary power in the average human life, and their impulses are great in the family and the business of life. The end of this second period is marked clearly in the female menopause.

In the third period mental interests begin to prevail, and show themselves in the practical mental guidance of emotional interests. As Emerson remarked, if there is marriage in later life the parties thereto usually have an eye on the cupboard. The grandmother—in this stage—can be more useful to the grandchildren by providing their parents with knowledge than by being another mother, and perhaps even very emotionally so.

Now, coming to our main topic in the consideration of these stages of life, that is, to old age, what have we to say? There is the decline of the senses, and of the active powers of the body. There is no decline of the mind, if it has been used—if the first three periods have been properly lived. There is now a state of mind in which not action, nor emotion, nor mental appraisal is the prevailing activity, each obscuring the other two to some extent while the special lesson of the period is being learned— just as in school arithmetic is set aside in the history period and *vice versa*. There is now a new kind of evaluation, in which action, emotion and mentality all have their equal and mature synthesis. It is not suggested that the subject is aware of this, but that this is the process which now sets in and provides the impulse for this current of life.

I have a very striking example of this in my collection of memories. This was the case of my own father, when he was up in his eighties or nineties. As a youth and a young man he had spent about eight years in sailing ships going to far parts of the earth. In his later age he used frequently to speak about those early experiences. One day my younger brother said to him, "Why are you always bothering about those old ships? Surely many more important things have happened recently." "Well," he replied, "the fact is that they mean so much more to me now than they did then."

The decline of the senses and active powers of the body is concomitant with this ripening of the mind and this fruitage of experience. Shall we then lament the condition of old age, or shall we not rather say that here too we have something very valuable preserved and increased in the most advanced organisms —the humans, that is?

In this case, truly, the benefit is not handed on by heredity, but it is handed on by social contact as far as such inward human synthesis and ripening can be handed on.

This chapter may well conclude with a few words about the value of material experience, and the curious fact that life advances by voluntary self-limitation. It is at once the paradox of life and the secret of its advancement.

In living we humans are not merely passive recipients of experience from outside. On the contrary we are always doing something about it—making decisions, seeking those things which give us agreeable feelings and avoiding others that have the reverse effect, using our brains to plan and select as far as our power and knowledge permit. These impulses we usually classify as thinking, liking or loving, and willing, all of which begin with one thing in common—a restriction.

You become interested in a cow in a field. You stop to pay special attention to it. Immediately you have narrowed or restricted the field of attention. But this act of reduction of *quantity* of intake into consciousness results in an accretion of *quality*. The clarity and strength of the conscious experience is enhanced by this act of concentration, as it is often called. More than that, there is also an increase of *power,* so that when that consciousness operates again in the same field of its activity it is clearer and stronger than it was before. There is also a specific gain with reference to the appreciation of sounds, or colors, or shapes, for example, so that those things are henceforth taken into consciousness with more clarity and strength—more truth, that is. There is also increased conscious power, surety of aim, grip of conscious perception on the object of sense, or on the thought of it. In short, there is growth, just as there is in a muscle of the arm, which may have been exercised for ten minutes in the morning with the aid of dumbells or bar-bells or something else, and yet the strength gained by that is afterwards available all day for the lifting of boxes or bags.

This law of *recuiller pour mieux sauter* is only the first part of an act of thinking. It is followed by expansion, for now we put two things (or more) together, and compare and classify them, noting their similarities or points in common, and their differences. "Yes, one is a white cow and the other a red cow." Certainly, but our red must be very red and verily red, our white must be very white and verily white, and our cow very cow and verily cow—verities which have to be gained by specific attention.

The law is that the gain of quality and clarity and power, acquired by the act of concentration, is available now for the act of expansion or inclusion. But it must be attended to and used. The data of attention must be clear, strong and valid; every bit of it should ring like a bell and be of good tone.

This law, which is fundamental in thinking—that is, in the thinking department of our conscious living—is true in our loving or goodwill also. That, too, grows by specific attention to it. So, in the second stage of life, properly directed by love, including interest in things, there is contraction or concentration on a specific object at a given time—a person, an animal, a flower, an idea. And just as in the case of attention to colors or sounds there is an increased imbibing or higher quality of conscious experience and also conscious awakening to an increased state and sense of being, so in the case of love there is new clarity and strength in the concentration, which can be retained in the following expansion or inclusion: Surely I love my wife better if I have loved my mother, and I love my children better if I have loved my wife, and I love my friends better because I have loved these three. Or else, let me beware! I may be drifting through life; I may be loving without proper attention, just as some people go through life only half-breathing.

It is of the essence of love that it must be love. Like the word of the Quaker, whose yea is yea and his nay nay, our love has to be true love or else it is not love at all. Only purity is possible here, as only truth is possible in thought. And let us be aware of our love and our thought. In my thinking it is for me to face my problem or my student task, and pause and say to myself, "I must think about this," and so in my loving problem or my studentship of loving (mainly in family life) it is well that I should pause occasionally and say, "I must love about this," and ask myself, "How much love is here, and how much adulteration." It is true that an adulterous individual or an adulterous generation seeketh for a sign, where there is no signpost; only the driver knows this road.

What is true of thought and love is the law also in the matter of making decisions. This also grows by exercise, so one cannot think for another, or love for another, to the detriment of that other's freedom of decision, if there is to be growth in this field, or in the particular concerned, in which authority or force may, unfortunately, have to be exercised. The act of will, too, begins with a specification.

The upshot of this relationship between any one of us and the world is that we gain from everything; in one way or another there is enrichment for us in everything that catches our eye. The world is incredibly valuable to us—every bit of it. What paucity of being would be ours—a veritable nothing—without all this. Truly that was a great symbolism which said, "Take and eat ye all of this," eat indeed the living bread, the bread of life, and receive in yourself—at your end of the line—the awakening which is never lost.

Chapter 5

Emotional Pain

How many people have stopped to look at the simple fact that we do not have pain in dreams? Consider all those nightmares or near-nightmares, in which everything is going wrong, the walls are falling in on us, the bogey-man is about to jump upon our backs. Imagination fails in recalling those grim experiences, but in none of them did anyone experience any pain. It is not that these dreams lack reality. They are as vivid, surely as our daily experience. Sit down, close your eyes and make a mental picture of something—a pair of scissors or a teapot. What a poor simulacrum it is; but those scissors seen in a dream are as real and true as if you saw them with your eyes. Yet they give no actual pain, not even if someone in the dreadful drama sticks them into your eyes.

We are incapable of imagining pain. It cannot get into our minds as it gets into our flesh. We cannot even recall pain in our memory.

I have spoken about actual pain, but not of emotional pain. Emotional pains we have in abundance in those dreams, and also in our waking imaginings. Fear is one of them, with all its brood of anxieties, misgivings, alarms, apprehensions, phobias, dreads, consternations, dismays, terrors, panics, shocks and horrors. Anger is another, with its embitterments. Pride a third, with its irritations, resentments, indignations, animosities, arrogances, frustrations and thwarted egotism.

We may safely say that the amount of actual pain in an average day of life, whether in animal or man, is small as compared with the amount of pleasure—I refer of course to the simple pleasures which accompany our common actions of living, not too conspicuous, exciting or outstanding pleasures looked forward to as belonging to special occasions, such as Christmas, or the expected results of special and perhaps prolonged labors and efforts. This is true of the amount of actual pleasure compared with the amount of actual pain. But when we compare the emotional pleasures and pains the picture is reversed. The amount of pleasurable emotion in an average person on an average day is far, far less than the amount of painful emotion.

We see this reflected in literature, in poetry and the epics, as well as in the problem novels of our day. It is not so with the animals; they show alertness as a primary instinct, though not usually accompanied by fear. And yet fear belongs properly to the animals, and is tremendously useful to them on the special occasions when extra fighting is necessary, or swifter flight, at which time it can spur and arm the animal into greater efforts by its call upon the reserves of the adrenal glands. But civilized man, sitting in his office and reading the stockmarket reports, can be full of fear and anxiety which, alas, will call his adrenal reserves into action when there is no fight, or flight, much to the detriment of his bodily health.

So much, indeed, is all our thinking permeated by emotional pain that we can find a Shelley writing "Our sincerest laughter with some pain is fraught." Consider also the implication of the well known line: "Man looks before and after, and longs for what is not."

The poet Robert Burns perhaps most clearly expressed the distinction between men and animals in this respect, in his well-known *Ode to a Field Mouse:*

> Wee, sleekit, cowrin', timrous beastie,
> Oh, what a panic's in thy breastie!
> Thou needna start awa' sae hasty,
>   Wi' bick'ring brattle!
> I wad be laith to rin and chase thee,
>   Wi' murd'ring pattle!
>
> But Mousie, thou art no thy lane
> In proving foresight may be vain!

> The best-laid schemes o' mice and men
>   Gang aft a-gley,
> And lea'e us nought but grief and pain
>   For promised joy.
>
> But thou art blest, compared wi' me!
>   The present only toucheth thee:
> But, och! I backward cast my e'e
>   On prospects drear!
> And forward, though I canna see,
>   I guess and fear.

Shakespeare expressed one aspect of the same sentiment in one of his grand and thunderous sonnets:

> When I have seen by Time's fell hand defaced
> The rich-proud cost of outworn buried age;
> When sometime lofty towers I see down-razed,
> And brass eternal slave to mortal rage;
> When I have seen the hungry ocean gain
> Advantage on the kingdom of the shore,
> And the firm soil win of the watery main,
> Increasing store with loss and loss with store;
> When I have seen such interchange of state,
> Or state itself confounded to decay;
> Ruin hath taught me thus to ruminate,
> That Time will come and take my love away.
>   This thought is as a death, which cannot choose
>   But weep to have that which it fears to lose.

I do not recollect that any of these poets ever offered us an antidote to this miserable state of mind. But Buddha in old India, although he spoke about our piteous plight as strongly as anybody, did offer a solution. So did the Stoics in Greece.

One trouble is to hold onto more possessions than one can conveniently handle. It is true that where there is possession there is the prospect of loss, where there is desire there is the prospect of failure, where there is fear there is the prospect of indignity and where there is error—to which all are prone—there is prospect of calamity.

Thus, even when there is no trouble there is often the thought of trouble, and there is anxiety about it. I live near some streets of suburban bungalows where many young children are to be seen playing together on the lawns. They are happy in the enjoyment of their limbs and senses, and they give great happiness to such as me, who have the pleasure of seeing them at play. The children have no anxieties, but the mothers who are busy behind those doors, and keep on popping out occasionally, are troubled by possible accidents and hurts. There is the oft-mentioned case of the mother whose child actually did meet with an accident. In the midst of her sorrow she said, "I knew something was going to happen this morning." What she did not stop to remember was that she had had similar anxiety every morning when the child went out to play.

Having mentioned the widespread Western view of the so-called pessimism of Buddha, I must now in fairness say that it was he who also described life as "wonderful, dear and pleasant unto each" when he was persuading King Bimbisara not to sacrifice goats and sheep on his altars. In simple justice, after quoting as I have, I must emphasize that Buddha cannot be accused of pessimism, for the reason that after stating that life is full of troubles he added that it need not be so. He said: "Ye suffer from yourselves," and further, he made the suffering quite definitely an individual problem.

It was emphatically a case of, "You, John Doe, suffer from yourself,"—not a collective affair. Further, still addressing the individual, he spoke of the way to the cessation of suffering as a proper mode of life, including correct understanding, views, outlook, appraisal, judgment, aims, motives, plans, considerations, decisions, speech, behavior, conduct, actions, livelihood, effort, intellectual activity, and contemplation.[3]

These he called the Path, and maintained that not only would the end of it be undiluted happiness, but also that its joy would soon in a very large measure reflect itself backwards, so to say,

[3] For details, see *Great Systems of Yoga,* by Ernest Wood. Pub. by Philosophical Library, Inc., New York.

onto the Path itself. Addressing the individual he exhorted him:
> Enter the Path! There spring the healing streams
>   Quenching all thirst! There bloom th' immortal flowers
> Carpeting all the way with joy! There throng
>   Swiftest and sweetest hours![4]

There were, in his eyes, two causes at work in producing this carpeting with joy. There was first the life of absolutely unqualified goodwill, which more and more puts one in harmony with others and, to say the least, removes from the mind all feelings of hatred and antagonism. Incidentally, it eliminates also most of the common human conflicts to which such feelings give rise.

The second cause of joy on the way was the belief in the "Law of Good."

He held very strongly a theory of material causation (which has been translated usually by the term "dependent origination") by which he maintained that in the changes around us in the world everything that happened was the cause of what followed, and nothing was self-caused but all forms originated in this dependent way. He was so much in line with the principle of causality so fundamental nowadays in modern science that he included the mind and its thoughts in this stream of causation. Care is to be taken here not to attribute the character or reactions of the mind to material objects. The meaning clearly was that minds with *their* qualities (just as, let us say, iron with *its* qualities) were a part of the unbroken continuum.

Buddha went still further and affirmed that goodness or justice was also to be included, or, as we might today express it, in our relationship with one another there is some law which is as automatic and calculable as the balance of attractions and separations which occur in nature under the law of gravitation. Indeed it is argued that no feeling for the welfare of another, no "good Samaritan" impulse, could possibly have arisen in any human being unless it was part of nature, a definite ingredient of our constitution which, like thought, is found to grow by

[4]*The Light of Asia,* by Sir Edwin Arnold.

encouragement and use. Under this law, there is justice in the world, and the condition of our ceasing to receive hurt from others is that we cease to give hurt to them.

This belief, which was widespread in India even before the time of Buddha, and today is being strongly affirmed by the modern Theosophists on its merits—not as a creed—has also another side to it. It goes along with the idea that if you do an injury to another there is a cause for it, there is a deficiency in your character. It may be a lack of perception of what that other is feeling, due to lack of interest in that feeling, due in turn to too much preoccupation with one's own separate or selfish desires.

If this is the case, and there is truth in this idea of the Law of Good, or Justice, we may infer that the person who is suffering at the hands of others is being educated by that. He is having "a dose of his own medicine," and afterwards the feeling of it will arise in himself when he sees similar suffering in another, and thereby the impulse of fellow feeling will grow.

This impulse so widely developed in human beings and increasing all the time, is surely not what one materially inclined scientist called "a beautiful disease," out of tune with the laws of evolution.

On these several grounds Buddha's view of life could be regarded as one of the greatest optimism, and his advice could be summed up in a few words, "Live without harming others, and regard all trouble from others as payment of your debts—overpay, if you can." The law will not allow overpayment, of course.

Possibly Jesus was also thinking of the idea that our misfortunes are valuably educative when he told the disciples that the Father knew of what they had need, and emphasized the lesson by stating that even though two sparrows are sold for a farthing, "One of them shall not fall on the ground without your Father," —presumably the almighty ever-presence of the first Principle or Uncaused Cause, whose presence must be law, since it was declared to be operative always and everywhere.

The principle of growth through action and experience is everywhere seen in nature. And everywhere also growth is found to be a pleasure—or at least expansion or enhancement of faculty or sense of life is so found to be. The mentality of man comes within the same category. It is part of life and its activity as such is a pleasure. Even the lugubrious person who is intent upon his own ailments and misfortunes is enjoying himself with his expansion of his knowledge of them or of his ego. He may think he isn't, but why does he do it? In living it seems there is always growing and always something that we like.

There is constantly with us this overtone of the joy of being, which no doubt stems from the self that we *are,* which evidently is much better and wiser than the self which we *think*. Our thinking obviously lags behind our being. The function of thinking which clearly has the purpose of enabling us to find our way about among the things of the world, seems quite inefficient when it is turned inward beyond the objective—beyond the body and even the mind itself. It is well, is it not, that among the birds and squirrels there is so much of being and so little of knowing. We see them enjoying themselves without thinking about it. It seems, in fact, that knowing about the living would take the edge off it in their case. Their knowledge has to do with things, and is of no value in itself—just as with us a spade or a piano has no use in itself, but has value only for digging or music. Thus an animal has need to know only what it needs to know—not to know the knowing—for its action is itself pleasurable, and its pleasure is in the actions of its being. An animal needs to know only what it needs to know, but does not need to know that it has knowledge, though when the application of that knowledge is obstructed there is pain. Even then the pain is beneficial. It arouses hidden reserve and the animal thereupon fights the obstruction, or else, with more careful observation, or with recognition of the obstruction as something dealt with before, it proceeds not to fight but to circumvent the obstacle. In the latter case—to be brief—the animal, instead of trying to change the object, changes itself. The fox, seeking hens, does not fight the wall that stands in his way; he seeks a hole in it, or he climbs over it. Thus he develops himself, and finds new activity and enjoyment, additional to the enjoyment of eating hens.

From the time when I first came to know about the little paramecium I have had unbounded admiration for it. This little animal swings towards its food, and sometimes misses it and bumps its nose on something else. At once it backs off a little way, turns a trifle on the axis of its own body length—changes direction, that is—and aims again for the new angle. Why that change of angle? This is not caused by any part of its environment. It is an example of the change of itself, as distinguished from fighting against something else, which stubbornly resists or repels it with force.

In this view there is a perception that it is matter, not life, that fights, paradoxical as the statement may seem. That piece of rock stands there and resists any intrusion by others upon the space which it has appropriated and in which it is (relatively speaking) sitting still. Strike the rock with your bare fist and you will see which of you gets most hurt—the man or the rock.

Even in the fight in which the man overcomes the rock with the aid of tools, the man is largely adapting himself, not the rock. In this fight he becomes the servant of his tools. He develops his arm and shoulder, and uses his hand as a socket for holding the tool with which he applies force to the rock. Then consider the woman—by contrast—who has had little to do with rocks, but much to do with delicate and thoughtful operations such as sewing, and here you find that it is the fingers which have grown deft and fine. It is with respect to such fineness that we men come to regard women as more related to life, more spiritual, even in their bodies, than we are, and so the deft fingers, the small waist and the delicate feet that pick their way rather than clump fightingly along the road have come to be not only a matter of admiration but also of inspiration to us who look on wonderingly. Indeed, one may go so far as to say that the female ovum is far more intelligent or alive than the male spermatozoon. A thousand of those blind blunderers are needed for every one that fulfils its purpose in one ovum.

While Buddha said, "Ye suffer from yourselves," another, older —how old we know not—philosophy of India, entitled the Sānkhya, opened its theme by stating that man suffers from three things, namely, (1) material objects, (2) other living beings and (3) himself. He also gets pleasure from the same three sources—indeed he gets two benefits, one from seeing in the world excellencies of which he would not otherwise become aware, and the second from using his thought, his feelings and his will in dealing with them. We learn, as the expression is, from all we see in nature. Or rather, when we see the things around us, especially the living things, there is a response in ourselves, which is of the nature of an awakening.

Buddha, we find, recommended knowledge about the mind and its ways, as a cure for the mind's ills and pains. The Sānkhya philosophy, of which I now speak, had the same recipe or prescription.

The name Sānkhya means knowledge, or at least classification, which comes to much the same thing. The first division of the universe, according to this philosophy, is into spirit and matter *(purusha* and *prakriti).* Included under matter was everything connected with both body and mind. Now, in order to compare or even to distinguish between spirit and matter one must know them both. It is not enough to say that spirit is that which is not matter. If, then, you can clearly distinguish between matter and spirit your problem of suffering is solved, because you thereby know the spirit, or the life. And if you know the spirit you know that it is impregnable, and you find yourself aligned with that.

Their word for the spirit *(purusha)* was one which means literally the dweller in the body, the body being referred to as a city *(puri)* because of its complex character. It is interesting to note a similarity of outlook (or is it inlook?) in the famous *Bhagavad Gita,* in which it speaks of the life or spirit as the "owner" of the body *(dehin),* not even the "dweller" in the body, and thereby creates and asserts the idea that a man is not a prisoner or refugee in the body but the user of the body for the purposes of the owner, himself. In this idea, when it is dwelt upon and clearly seen, there is a special value to the psychiatrist or mental healer. The Sānkhyas were and are very clear about this. They say that it is not you, the *purusha,* who is suffering, but it is the infirmities of your bodies (body and mind) that are reflected into you. It is, I think, much as if an artist were so wrapped up in his picture that he would be terribly distressed by its defects. Those defects in us are pains in the body and mind.

In this connection let us consider that bodily health is a feeling in the body when its organs and functions are all in harmonious activity. When some disharmony occurs — through accident, wrong food and insufficient or excess exercise or rest—there is pain, and pain is an indication that there is something which needs to be put right. It is then, the height of folly to try to get rid of pain without understanding what is wrong and doing something about that. Physically, it is some obstruction to the smooth natural working of the body, some blocking or distortion of its natural free flow which gives rise to pain. It is known also that unnatural emotions and thoughts also cause disorder in the body, giving rise to pain.

It was the same philosophers, the Sānkhyas, who put forward the statement that in nature there are three modes of relationship—(1) the inert or resistive, (2) the forceful or aggressive, and (3) the adaptable or harmonious. The last is the key of growth or evolution, not only growth in size, but in complexity or organization.

The inert person resists change, the aggressive wants change, the harmonious wants a proper use of these two in the balance of the old and the new which is what we know as harmonious living. Our life at any given moment must be partly old and partly new. If it were nothing but a repetition of the past there would be none of that growth or increase which is felt as living. If it were all new we would not be ourselves for two successive moments. The balance or poise of life is a dynamism in the static and a static in the dynamism. The choice of how much of the past we will adhere to or repeat in the present, and how much it shall be altered is intelligence. The balanced life is the healthy and happy one. It is a matter of poise between the past and the future, like the poise of a runner or a dancer. The runner must not, and in fact cannot outrun himself; he must take himself with him. The whole universe exemplifies these three fundamental or ever present characteristics. Its essential peace —there is no fundamental destruction in nature—may be disturbed here and there by a spot or lump too inert or too aimlessly active, but the third principle, or balance, will soon bring in its corrective influence. Life is superior to space and time. Space-facts (material forms) and time-facts (intellections) are only its servants.

It is very interesting to observe that everything aims at peace. Even the storm does so. This is my favorite example—a storm at sea. We are on a ship, gliding smoothly on a placid ocean beneath a calm blue sky with a few white clouds. But what is this? A gust of wind strikes us. We look whence it comes. A dark, black cloud appears. It is getting heavier and descending, driving the air before it. Soon we are in the midst of an uproar—tossing turbulent waves and violent winds, perhaps lightning and thunder. Then comes the rain, in a heavy torrent, beating down and flattening the waves. The wind is no more. Soon the rain also is no more. The sun is shining again, and again the sea and sky are serene, enjoying as it were their gentle interchange of being. That dreadful violence was only aiming at peace; it was a restoration from an unbalance, a relief from a strain in the atmosphere, where something had lagged. Or we could take the example of a volcano—but there is no need to elaborate. The lesson of nature is obvious; everywhere all violence is aiming at peace.

Be it so, also, then, in that little universe which is a man, and in the interests of happiness and peace let him have the intelligence to know when forcefulness, aggressiveness and change are proper and when they are not. Let this be applied to human life and then in the midst of it all and participating in it, we may attain the peace of strength, not the peace of protectedness. This mode of living was evidently aimed at by Reinhold Niebuhr, Professor of Ethics at the Union Theological Seminary, New York, when he formed the following prayer:

> Give me the serenity to accept what cannot be changed;
> Give me the courage to change what must be changed;
> The wisdom to distinguish one from the other.

Chapter 6

The Value of Emotional Pains

The best way to reduce the amount of pain in a human life is to recognize its great value as a signpost of the wrong way, and then to study and correct the errors or defects which it indicates. One might say: "Do not invite pain; but welcome it when it comes."

It is, of course, best to be alert in the matter of pain as animals are alert. How the birds in the garden all fly up, if I give so much as a flick to the window curtain! It is not in fear, I think, that they so fly, but just as a part of the alertness of life. They go up there on the railing or in the trees, and will all be down and busy eating again before long, their little hearts as sound as a bell, as before. No doubt the interlude had its value also, for it cannot be good even for them to be eating all the time!

The human being has to be alert with all his faculties, to avoid pains. "His faculties" means mostly the mental. In the conditions of complexity of the modern home there are many reasons for alertness. So be alert; be cautious. Indeed statistics show that there are more serious accidents in the homes of the people than in the roads among the motorcars, with all their dramatic daily toll of deaths and injuries.

Among intelligent people this alertness need not become in itself a pain. It is not a trouble; it is living (Rejoice, O my heart!) and need not contain the slightest trace of fear or anxiety. But did I not read in the paper this morning that Mr. A. fell off a ladder and broke both legs and an arm? Yes, and I know also that he must have (a) used a defective ladder, (b) placed it crookedly, or (c) leaned over too far—one, two or three of these—and all due to laziness on his part. Or perhaps it was due to (d) worry about something else—perhaps nothing better than annoyance at having to do this job. This man had better just sit down and think a bit—preferably before the event, but anyhow afterwards. Yes, think and think, until he learns the joy of living—the joy of just living. "But I want to be out and playing golf, and here I am fixing this paint or wall-paper." "So, and how did you get yourself into that position, my friend?" "Don't 'friend' me,"—he grinds his teeth—"but look at your own mess." On this note of camaraderie, we adjourn the meeting until the next visit.

Meantime, my friend—he really *is* that—frets and fumes, unless he can distract himself with the novel I have sent him, or with a pretty nurse. He frets and fumes, and so he has *double trouble*—the real pains of his injuries, and the emotional pains which he is piling up on top of them. Double trouble is only too mild a title for this emotional condition. "Be on guard, my friend (O, why must I say that again?) against the double trouble," I admonish him, in parting. He turns to the nurse, "How can one tolerate this irritating blighter?" he complains. "I hope he will not come again." But he knows, and I know, and perhaps the nurse knows, that at any moment he would rush to save my life, at the risk of his own.

I suppose we could make a long list of the many kinds of double trouble including the very familiar forms of anxiety and worry. These emotions are harmful in several ways. The only way in which they are useful is in their painfulness—these pains could warn us that there is something wrong which should be studied and dealt with. The harm is that they waste time, dissipate energy, deplete vitality and not only divert thought but positively destroy it.

These emotional troubles are not only thus damaging to the day's richness of living—which is, as I have pointed out, the enjoyment of the use of one's faculties of body and mind in relation to the successive events of the day. They have also two other main forms of destructiveness—psychosomatic effects, and social disharmony or crime.

These psychosomatic conditions are not merely imaginary ailments, but are—as I suppose most people know nowadays—actual bodily disorders, including proneness to infection, brought on by the emotional conditions we have been considering. The volume of this kind of human trouble was brought forcibly to my attention one day while I was strolling in the grounds of a large state hospital along with one of its senior doctors. I was much impressed by the size of the pile of buildings, and the almost fantastic number of windows presented to my view. I commented on the vast collection of pain and trouble behind those windows. "Yes," remarked my companion, "and do you know that more than seventy-five per cent of the cases are psychosomatic?"

Two far-reaching effects of the same cause are to be frequently seen in various forms of insanity and criminality also. That anxiety can not only poison the day and unseat the power of reason to deal with the feared event, but positively drive a person into psychoses which dominate the mind's attention constantly even when there is no actual material cause for anxiety —the same being perhaps imaginary, perhaps exaggerated, perhaps gone—is well known. That this is a potent cause of untruthfulness, one of the chief causes of the mutual mistrust which spoils so much of our social contact is not so often noticed. Long ago Shakespeare drew pointed attention to it in *Henry the Fifth,* where the king, pointing out to the Earl of Cambridge the enormity of his treasonable offence, went beyond his personal concern and said:

> Such and so finely bolted didst thou seem:
> And thus thy fall hath left a kind of blot,
> To mark the full-fraught man and best indued
> With some suspicion. I will weep for thee;
> For this revolt of thine, methinks, is like
> Another fall of man.

The psychosis of anxiety sometimes builds up to the point of madness, in which it thrusts itself forward on all sorts of inappropriate occasions, and even in bad cases almost all the time, because of its cumulative effect, or habit. It is liable to sink below the surface of attention and gain a major footing in that collection of mental habits, which is often called the subconscious mind. I like the term "subconscious mind" better than the term "unconscious mind" here, because it draws attention to the fact that at some time the error or trouble was within the field of conscious attention and now has fallen below it. That it should extrude or upthrust itself so strongly and frequently is not in itself a defect, but is merely an example of the regular procedure of the stream or drift of ideas, which is sometimes called uncontrolled thought, but is really no thought at all, but the drift of memories.

It is well-known, I believe, that in common dreaming (which is not thought, but a drift of uncontrolled ideas) we never experience anything completely new to us, such as is possible in waking life. All such dream occurrences are the flowing along and interweaving (not logical or creative combination) of the contents of the lower mind. I like to use this expression "lower mind" at this point because of the prevalence of waking or conscious drift, which people sometimes mistake for thought when they express an opinion which is by no means a piece of current thinking, but only an emergence from the past. As to the occasional new and true experiences during sleep, these are real extrasensory perceptions, or else impressions from the higher mind, not dreamings.

What happens in this "lower mind" is quite natural and orderly. Events and ideas have entered into that collection of memories and stand there most strongly when they have been either repeated many times or been thrust into it with a violent impact. As an example of the latter: someone may mention the intersection of Fifth Avenue and Forty-second Street. Instantly jumps up from your "lower mind," or mental museum, or whatever we may call it, the picture of a motorcar accident you had there twenty years ago.

In the dream or drift of daydreaming one idea or picture succeeds another not haphazardly but because of a mental relationship of one kind or another (what I have called "roads of thought"), according to the principle of greatest facility or that of violent impact. The anxiety which becomes a psychosis is therefore following the natural course of things. It has become a psychosis, perhaps to the point of insanity, ousting all reason, one's own and that of other people who may try to help, because of its repetition or its original impact.

Have we here depicted some kind of a pain which is not useful? This insanity has natural utility in that it certainly would make for quick elimination from the ranks of the living, were the person not maintained and protected by other people. But in what way does it benefit the individual most concerned? Thus we know that a sensible person, finding an anxiety in his mind, and recognizing it as an emotional trouble, will bring forth all the thinking of which he is capable, judge the degree of probability of the real danger (if any) and relegate it to its proportional allowance of attention in the scheme of daily living, in which hazards are unavoidable by emotional means and calculated risks are part of the valuable stimulation of living. If in the earlier stages of an anxiety the subject will not take the trouble to face the facts of outward life and inward emotion mentally and deal with them mentally or consider the value of the advice given to him by parents, teachers, and friends including books, in this connection, he must expect the anxiety to increase. Anxiety has no use in human life, except, as in the case of other pains, as an indicator of danger, and if taken as such as an awakener of more intelligent activity and growth. If this is neglected, the lesson may be expected to become more and more severe.

It is at this point that we must introduce another factor—the ego. Further on we will see what part this plays in these emotional psychoses. In the meantime let us notice that the anxiety is sometimes, nay often, fostered by the subject of it, because it fosters a spurious build-up of self-importance. There is no question about the validity and value of what I would call "the self-experience of unity," but the dangers and emotional pains of the spurious ego-pictures or self-images which abound are tremendous.

Of these more anon, but let us at least now notice that these emotions also are prolific sources of insanity, and sometimes of psychosomatic disorders and diseases.

When my doctor friend told me that at least three quarters of the cases in his huge hospital were psychosomatic, I found myself responding with great enthusiasm: "Isn't that heartening, for we know very well how to correct the mind, though we do not know very well how to correct the body." I was thinking that in curing even small bodily ailments, we often must have recourse to special exercises, or to some special herbs or chemicals outside the regular course of nutrition, but in the case of the mind the cure is contained in itself. I think my psychiatrist friends will confirm this statement to the extent that in very many cases—I may say the majority of cases?—the psychiatric doctor is not trying to introduce something new into the patient's mind, nor to persuade him to accept any theory or belief, but rather simply to bring about a condition in which the patient will see for himself the cause of his trouble, and then the knowledge so revealed will be to some extent, or even entirely, curative.

But my pleasure at the news was further fed by another consideration. I had made such a long and detailed study of many time-honored ways of dealing with the emotions before they became so bad as to need the help of a psychiatrist that I was confident that all that people needed in order to avoid the psychosomatic condition described by my doctor friend was some general education (preferably in schools and colleges) about the nature of the emotions and the workings of the mind—which, alas, is very conspicuously lacking at present.

It may be remarked that I am propounding a system of prophylaxis, or preventive knowledge. Just so, but not that alone; one that is also curative in all cases where the emotional disease has not gone too far. I have remarked that a large part of human thought is given to precautions of various kinds, while another part is engaged in creative planning. Let us have as big a proportion of precautionary knowledge with reference to the emotions as we have with regard to material activities, and great benefit will I am sure very soon ensue.

Let me now give some time-honored studies along these lines in another chapter.

Chapter 7

The Cure of Emotional Pains

In our last chapter I have spoken of knowledge as the cure for emotional pains, whether that knowledge be due to general informative education, or to investigation and thinking on the part of the sufferer or of a psychological doctor, or either of them helped by the other. The general principle of the developmental function of pain in the evolutionary process holds good. It is a function, of course, of a negative kind, inasmuch as the evolution takes place through efforts to eliminate specific pains. Let us briefly review it.

The pain of hunger goads primitive organisms into their hit-and-miss efforts to get food, the getting leads to pleasure, excess pleasure leads to pain again, and this leads in turn to the development of thought. Thought is used then to guide action and feeling into paths favorable to the natural welfare and health of the organism. The mental process is next seen to have its own form of pleasure, and also to lead to pain again, internal pain when it discovers that it cannot grow to immense capacity—just as the body cannot grow to immense stature and strength—and external pain when it serves excess pleasure which leads to bodily disorders or to fights and wars—either greedy or fanatical. This new pain paves the way for ethical knowledge and ethical feeling (love of lives) to grow, especially when the mentality yields to that interest and motive and serves it.

In their treatment of pain (individual miracles aside—a drop in the bucket of pains) Jesus and Buddha laid nearly all their emphasis on ethical development. Jesus insisted above everything else —although giving many pieces of good advice on minor matters— that the way to happiness was through the practice of love. The famous two commandments: love of God and love of neighbor, will be recalled by all in this connection.

Jesus did, however, bring out some striking psychological statements, very much in line with modern thought. For example: "Either make the tree good, and (thereby) his fruit good; or else make the tree corrupt, and his fruit corrupt; for the tree is known by his fruit . . . out of the abundance of the heart the mouth speaketh. A good man out of the good treasure of the heart bringeth forth good things: and an evil man out of the evil treasure bringeth forth evil things . . . every idle word that men shall speak, they shall give account thereof . . ."[6] This pronouncement with its statements about *making* the tree and its reference to idle words comes rather near to the idea of the subconscious mind as a museum or treasury of our past.

It is to be noted that when Jesus said, "Make the tree good" he was addressing the people, and he preceded the entire statement by, "I say unto you," indicating that they were the makers for themselves of what I have compared with the subconscious mind.

Quite in line with this is that often-criticized portion of the Lord's Prayer: "Lead us not into temptation." It is really good psychology, because we are all the time, or at least now and then, at work on that magma of our lower mind, or storage mind, or subconscious mind, bringing bits of it to the surface, cogitating them a little (even if not intentionally) and then returning them to their pigeon-holes or rather slots in that robot-mechanism of uncontrolled responses. That is one thing I am doing as I write this book, and you are doing as you read it. We are, I hope, making the tree better.

It is well, then, that what for us are temptations should be held back a bit until we are better able to handle them, for our ability to think *while* acting is also growing with exercise and use. There is of course, for us a nice balance all the time between action (doing) and thinking (turning experience over in our growing minds). Here lies another little useful problem: how much time we should give in each day to these two operations. I recollect the advice once given by an elderly successful business-man to a younger aspirant in that line. He said that he found that half an hour spent in the early morning considering all the business likely to come up

[6]Matthew: 12: 33-36.

during the day was not time wasted. It made that day much richer —some things were not overlooked or forgotten, in others he was not impulsively foolish, never did he get enthusiastic about something to the extent of neglecting caution or being impatient of cautiousness, and never did he over-fatigue himself by threshing about trying to decide what to do next, or how to fill spare time.

I have a keen memory of how pleased I was when I found that Patanjali had given his prescription on how to deal with undesired and incoming and uprising thoughts. He said: "Think to the contrary," (Aphorism ii 33) but immediately followed it by: "Thinking to the contrary is: 'The bad thought of injury, et cetera, whether done, caused to be done, or approved, whether preceded by greed, anger or infatuation, whether mild, or strong, results in endless pain and error.'" (Aphorism ii 34.) He did not recommend that elementary but wide-spread tendency to meditate on the opposite by substituting something "good" for something "bad," and assuming that the "bad" will die of inanition. Patanjali was a good psychologist, and his method was the method of nature. You do not make a better garden by planting more and more of what your present impulse leads you now to like, but you root out the bad, lest it come up in the night or the springtime, and you do not root it out by your present impulse or desire but after much thinking about it and seeing what it is and what it does.

Another very valuable psychological item indirectly contributed by Jesus was the expression, "Servants of sin." St. Paul used this expression very fully and strongly in his Epistle to the Romans: "Let not sin . . . reign in your mortal body . . . Neither yield ye your members unto sin . . . Know ye not that to whom ye yield yourselves servants to obey his servants ye are to whom ye obey . . . Even so now yield your members servants to righteousness . . . For when ye were the servants of sin, ye were free from righteousness. What fruit had ye then in those things whereof ye are now ashamed? for the end of those things is death."[7] The fact that in a further chapter Paul speaks of sin as the law of the flesh does not cancel out his prior statement that now in his enlightenment, "It

[7]*Op. cit.* Ch. 6.

is no more I that do it, but sin that dwelleth in me."[8]

The realization by a person that he himself is not sinful and does not originate sins, that he is not a sinner but only a servant of sin, is a powerful truth in the hands of the psychological healers belonging to several modern churches, such as the New Thought, the Church of the Science of Mind, and the Christian Scientist. This thought has proved itself a great refreshment and "release" to many people, even when accompanied, as sometimes, with the further thought that it is "the Christ in me," or that it is "the God within." In these two cases the man is visualizing himself as somewhere in the middle between the two, but in any case he is not the sinner. There is, of course, nothing to prevent members of other churches from seeing the value of this truth even if some of their preachers have not yet realized it.

A question has been put to me verbally as to why Jesus did not himself give the explanations which Paul gave. There are several reasons. First, he was preoccupied with the Law, the Prophets and the Messianic tradition. As a consequence he was primarily a messenger to the Jews. He was born among them physically and brought up among them emotionally and mentally. He quotes from the Jewish scriptures, and not a word from Socrates, Plato or Aristotle, or from the Stoics or the Greeks of Alexandria and other settlements. He seems to take seriously the Jehovan message given to Moses on Mt. Sinai, but accepts also the Prophets' insistence upon the direct judgment of each individual by God. He carries that individualism to its completion, and to the logical conclusion that his kingdom, promised in the prophesies, is not of this world.

He carries also his ethic beyond the idea that his message is for a special race of people, and asserts that it is for the whole world of men, without restrictions. He establishes no limited church, but says that his message, or bread from heaven, consists of the words of his doctrine. Still, to the day of his death he preached among the Jews and near-Jews, and mostly in immediate response to personal questions and the requirements of crowds or of his im-

[8]*Op. cit.* Ch. 7 vs. 17.

mediate disciples, who with two or three exceptions had little contact with Greek influence.

But Paul, though a Jew by race, was born a Greek by nationality, was acquainted with Greek and Greek-minded people, and showed much facility in handling psychological and metaphysical significances. He never deviated from Jesus' doctrines, but he was always presenting them to the Gentiles with a knowledge of the content and the workings of their minds. So much was this the case that the word Christian—a Greek word—was brought into use at first only at Antioch where Paul established his first center. Jesus did say his doctrine was for all men everywhere, but he left it to time, and to Paul—whom he personally instructed in the matter, according to Acts—to play a chief part in the spreading of it to the Gentiles. It is interesting that although the original disciples were sent out by Jesus they were to be guided in their work by the Holy Ghost, while Paul was directed from "the other world" by Jesus himself, according to Acts and Paul's belief.

Two well-known practical philosophies much concerned with the reaching of happiness by the avoidance of pain were widely spread in the Greek and Roman world around the Mediterranean —the Epicurean and the Stoic, both dating from about 300 B.C. It was while Paul was in Athens discoursing to some Stoics that he said that God had made of one blood all nations of men, and that all should seek him, "though he be not far from every one of us; for in him we live and move and have our being; as certain also of your own poets have said, for we are also his offspring."[9]

Both Epicureans and Stoics followed what in our day would probably be called a common-sense policy in personal life—adapt your life to the requirements of nature, and use your intelligence to help you in this policy. The difference between them was that the Epicureans proceeded to use reason more to guide them to a comfortable and healthy bodily existence, while the Stoics were more concerned with an austere control of emotions by reason, having observed that the follies and fancies of the mind are the chief cause of human trouble in the civilized world.

[9]Acts 17: 28.

An imaginary conversation between a Stoic and an Epicurean brings these differences clearly into view. The Stoic was visiting at the farm of the Epicurean. It was a well-ordered and placid scene, quite in accordance with the formula: "Do not poison the present with regrets for the past and fears for the future. Live a healthy well-ordered life and leave the rest to nature, which cannot be improved fundamentally by the art of man." The Stoic, however, drew attention to the important fact that if the mind is the source of our pain, it is also a means to great happiness, not only in its own working but also in its effects in life. The Stoic said, "Regard the process of nature concerning your valued possessions —your horses and houses and lands—do not these wither and decay when they are not constantly protected by the mind, and do you not constantly take thought for these things—their protection and preservation and improvement?" "Certainly," was the reply. "Well, then, what of your still more cherished possession, the mind? Does not this also require attention—proper nourishment and rest, and above all the exercise of its powers in all the business of life?"

There was another argument used to convince people of the fact that they really thought of themselves as the mind. If you go to a man and tell him that he is in an unhealthy condition, that his body seems to be out of order, and he had better consult a physician, he will take no offense; but if you approach the same man and say, "Look here, my friend, it seems to me that your mind is out of order. Your moral nature seems to be diseased. Do you not think you had better consult a psychologist or a priest?" he will at once become angry. There is no difference in the two cases, but that in the second you refer to the mind, not the body, and men feel themselves really touched when you refer to that. For many people, the mind is the ego.

So the Stoics established the idea that in the mind our happiness was to be sought. How, then, did they propose to get rid of pain without destroying happiness as well? This, they said, can be done by dividing your world into two parts. Study all things, and classify them as those which are within your power and those that are out of your power. Then, by allowing the mind to concern itself only with those that are within your power you will give it scope for activity and exercise, but not for distress or inquietude about any outside thing. To such an extent did the Stoics attain philosophical abstraction that they were able to put out of mind many things that would distress an ordinary man. There is the familiar example of the man thrown into prison who would consider that his body had now gone into the possession of his enemies, and he would trouble himself no more about it.

A story is told that the master of the Stoic Epictetus, of whose discourses there are excellent translations available, was a very strong man, and he sometimes amused himself at the expense of the philosopher. One day he was twisting Epictetus' leg, and the Stoic philosopher said to him, "Now if you twist that leg any more you will break it." The strong man did break the leg, but Epictetus did not trouble about it—the matter was outside his power.

The famous Roman senator Seneca, who along with many other leading men of the time was an adherent of Stoicism, gives us an example of the high ethical philosophy it contained. Speaking of a thief, he said that the man was a good man, and explained that he was good because he would much have preferred to obtain the stolen article honestly, but it was not possible and the temptation was too much for him. As to the occasional cases in which people delight in crimes, these will be fully discussed in our chapter on the egoistic emotions.

As regards these high sentiments about the nature of man, Epictetus went so far as to say: "There is only one thing for which God has sent me into the world, and that is to perfect myself in every sort of virtue, and there is nothing in all the world that cannot be used for that purpose." This carried the doctrine of non-resentment to its highest peak, but it did not propose that man should therefore be passive to the stream of events. The chief part of their usefulness lay in their presentation of matter for man's choice and treatment with reason and decision. So while a Seneca could choose the path of greatness in the world of politics, an Epictetus could choose the path of simplicity. So simple indeed was his life that when someone stole the brass vessel which stood near his doorway to hold his daily supply of water he could accept the situation without annoyance or regret, and say, "Oh well, the next time they come they will find at my door only a common earthern pot, not worth taking, and I shall rest in peace."

Chapter 8

The Egoic Pains

Of one thing I feel sure with regard to our human egoic pains—which play such an enormous and such a bitter role in modern psychology—they are growing pains. Just as bodily pains are linked with bodily development, and can perform the useful work of elimination of the unfit if they are not rightly received and attended to, and just as emotional pains have the same two functions, so also is the truth about egoic troubles. In all these cases, there is no "kill or cure," but there is always "grow or die." And just as natural bodily troubles are connected with the "grow or die" principle (hunger and food, cold and clothing, disease and natural immunity), so also are the troubles incident to the development of the self-image or the personality picture.

Was it not the great Goethe who, when asked to name the most prevalent and most consuming human desire, replied, "To be wanted"? I have no doubt that the complexes of desires enjoyed and suffered by birds and squirrels do not possess this element, which is born of the human mind. Some kinds of human crimes in which this item of development is very primitive or very deficient, are also of the animal kind, concerned only with bodily satisfactions and possessions. It is thus possible in the diagnosis of personal problems, to ask first whether the matter is one of the ego or not.

In an earlier chapter, in a brief study of the development of the mind of the human being, we have seen that in its early stages the human infant, while very highly conscious and sensitive and full of natural bodily reactions, has no personality-picture or ego-image. In fact, it has not even a knowledge of the "personality" or identity of anything. A primrose by the river's brink is not even a primrose to him. A breast is not to it a breast, or a mouth a mouth. The child is conscious. More, it is self-conscious. But it is not conscious of self. It is conscious of consciousness, without knowing this consciousness is its own. It very gradually distinguishes external things as such, then its own body as one of them, then that body as "of me." This is its *first mistake*. The consciousness is "of me," "mine," "my consciousness." The child mentally isolates itself from the environment, and identifies itself—first in animal fashion, by recognition, and afterwards in human fashion, by memory. Then, thinking itself to be that known thing, it comes to formulate "my consciousness."

This is no doubt a very profound error. According to the old Yoga and Vedanta schools of India it is the primal error *(avidyā)*, which is the cause of all our woe. According to Patanjali, the purpose of the Raja Yoga philosophy and practice of meditation is to control the ideas in the mind, especially this one, whereby the Looker (the self) will reside in his own proper nature, failing which he remains identified with the ideas.[10]

Pending, however, that consummation so devoutly to be desired, there are, says Patanjali, five sources of trouble. I will now list them as given in Aphorism ii 3: Possessiveness, aversion, desire, self-personality or egoism, and ignorance or error.[11] I have listed them here in reverse order, however, because that is the way in which they are overcome in the course of practice of Yoga philosophy. The most imprisoned man is he who can be hurt through his possessions. "Who am I? I am the man who lives at 45 Baker St., the house with the tulips in the garden." One lady told me that when she woke up in the morning it took her a moment to "realize who she was." This is true of all of us in some degree, as can easily be seen if we look into the matter. But sometimes she could not immediately identify herself, until she thought, "I am the woman who owns those three parrots."

A little self-analysis of this kind can be very helpful. It can loosen attachments to home, or even to nationality, through which

[10] *Yoga Sutras,* Aphorism i 2, 3.

[11] See *Practical Yoga: Ancient and Modern,* by Ernest Wood, E. P. Dutton & Co., New York.

we can easily be hurt. Sometimes it is bodily: "Alas, I am losing my beauty. Well, well, I still have my rocking chair."

One useful mode of release from these attachments is to consider what you would be without all these things, listing them one after another. Perhaps you dare not, because you have too many fears, or because you would feel "lost."

A second stage in this progress is that in which the person lives more or less "on the wing." If there is not one thing there will be some other thing, so it will be all right! Things are always changing; let us go along with what comes! But now, in these goings and comings of things, there are some that are liked and some that are disliked. These disliked ones are the things that have given pain in the past, so are now to be avoided. But there is more to it than that—there is association coming up from that storage mind. These people who have released themselves from the anchorage to possessions, are still in bondage to their established opinions and feelings about things. Some are hagridden by phobias of various kinds—the list is too numerous to mention.

One is perhaps in trouble in this way, when a friend comes along with a cheerful, "Let us look on the bright side." Then, appreciating the niceness of things, one wings one's way to something most desirable, or to too many. It is at this stage and the previous one that the pains and pleasures are emotional rather than physical. There is attachment to emotions. You care very much whether you are depressed or not. You are depressed about your depression, and so become doubly depressed. This is an example of an aversion to an aversion. Or, you are elated because you are elated; and once more anchored.

What releases from this bondage to emotional conditions? A mental view of them, and of this self of yours. You observe that after all you do not suffer and enjoy these things mainly according to what they are, but according to your opinion, which is perhaps not better than a subconscious prejudice against or for them. One has read of the case of the young woman in the psychology class who at last decided to marry the young man whose name was Norman, and what tipped the scales in his favor was her subconscious association of the name with normal. If his name had been Simeon he might have lost out, because of unconscious association with simian.

Perhaps in the last sentence I should not have written unconscious association but unmental or at least unobserved. When mental review of emotional attachments begins there is some release from them. But now there is egoity. "I am a man or mind with such and such possessions, and such and such emotional tendencies, and such and such thoughts about these things." Now, just as there is a comparison of thing and thing, and of emotion and emotion, and a judicious valuation and use of these, so there is a comparison of ego and ego—my ego and your ego, perhaps, or my miserably weak and handicapped ego as compared with what it might be. "Oh, how I would like to be liked by myself!" Here, so far from having a judicial knowledge of one's possessions and emotions, and of one's mind, one has a troubled mind, a troubled self-image, grasping, fighting, competing, for self-satisfaction with oneself. This can lead to some success, or to breakdown with subsequent death.

Perhaps the greatest blow to this self-appraisal, which even the successful have to face sooner or later is the realization of the puny possibility of even the best of human minds. You cannot, with a whole life-time's work, know much of many subjects, perhaps not all of any one science. So pride, love of one's own self-image, receives a shrewd blow. This ego cannot be blown up big, any more than the body can. Now all the brood of pride's ugly children begin to be dehydrated like jelly-fish on the beach. Will you then become a cynic saying, "At least I know."? Ha, ha, another pride, to self-satisfy this moribund self-image. You, James, you John, you wanted to sit on the right and left hand, much to the annoyance of the other ten disciples.

"Make no mistake," now pipes up Mr. Average Man, "I have no such notions of my own greatness, now or future." So: Let us go and have supper, and give thanks for our cooked food, and our good beds? No, sir, that won't do. All that egotism had its useful function. It brought that mentality to its full stature; even though that be less than the least in the kingdom of heaven.

The non-cynic will now say: "I see the way. Though man cannot be much, it is grand to be one of mankind. Mankind is great; let us have harmony, brotherly love, mutual help—from each according to his power, to each according to his need; each for all and all for each. I will be humble and satisfied with my little ego." No sir, that also won't do. I fear you will slack off—most people do once they reach the mature age of thirty-five or forty years (the age of deflation) and begin to realize that their youthful dreams of great success are doomed to failure. No sir, you need some pains or troubles. You are still, I fear, content with the avoidance of pain.

Let us be sure of one thing. The way to the ending of pain is the way of the worker, with no shadow of escapism and no "consolation philosophy." And with regard to these egoic pains the only proper treatment is to look them straight in the eye; examine each one of them as it arises. When you see what a fool thing that self-image is, it will die because you are not nourishing it any more. Otherwise, you are nourishing it with hope, almost perhaps a secret hope that "I"—this self-image—will find satisfaction. "Give up hope all ye who enter here;" for "Only the truth shall make you free." Get behind the self-image.

We have seen how possessiveness, antagonism, attachment and egoism gradually diminish in the order observed by Patanjali a few hundred years B.C. What trouble will now remain? The root of the egoism and the rest, namely *ignorance* about the self. "What am I?" is the question. All the self-images were found to be wrong, one after another, and the mind was kept at work on them by their inherent pain. Always the hunger; but now for self-realization.

When God was asked by Moses to describe himself, he said, "I am that I am."[12] This was not a mere putting off of the unready adherents or followers, as we can see if we read it with an emphasis on the second I: I am what *I* am—not what

[12]Exodus 3: 14.

something else is, not what the body is, or emotions are, or thought is or even love is, but what *I* am. I remember an occasion on which I was discussing this with a young man who was very eager to have the transcendental experience spoken of by the religious teachers of mankind and quite a number of people through the ages, when suddenly the young man caught the idea and exclaimed, "Why, Peter Piper (let this be his name) will *never* have that experience." I agreed with him and added, "But of course *you* will have it." That will become so when he gives up being "assimilated to the ideas." That realization will then be a matter of direct experience, but not of anything in any mental category.

The religious story about the descent into hell and rising on the third day is a good allegory. The mind of man is described as three-fold in the *Bhagavad Gita* and in the writings of Vedantists such as Shankaracharya. The *mind* of man, they say, has will, wisdom (which is love), and activity (which is thinking or thought). The last owns also a cellar in which it keeps the materials of its contact with the outer world (which is what I and many others have called the lower or subconscious mind). The whole mind is thus four-fold, but its own activity is three-fold, and the lower mind a sort of tomb. To say the best for it, the mind's activity always involves an occlusion, which is the daily and hourly experience of every one of us in the world. Very well, then, the three days are the three stages of progress in the overcoming of these limitations, the last of which contains the battle with the egoic pains.

Now let us look again at the alternations of bondage and release in every step of this progress or process of the mind; the descent, the overcoming and the ascent, in every single act of thought, however small. First the mind is subjected to some limited circumstances. You want to think about or study a cow; very well, you are excluding crabs and scorpions. You are taking in *some* factual material from the outside, through the senses, and then there is an act of withdrawal from and exclusion of further outside effects, and a study or consideration of the material already taken into the mind—in a word, thinking.

In this process of thinking there is the co-ordination of the information brought in by the different senses, and also there is the discovery of actions and relationships of the object (say, the cow) with others immediately connected with it and the internal relations of its parts in one coherent unity, comparable on a small scale with the invisible forces (such as gravitation) and laws (such as causality) which play such a great part in the unification or coherence of entire existence, or "the world."

This withdrawal into itself for the purposes of thinking is the very life of the mind, while its subjection to outside impact and influences is a sort of temporary death. If we were all the time bombarded by all the material from outside, without any letup, the mind would be completely obliterated. This last process is one of the techniques of brainwashing, and is also largely used in commercial advertising.

It will be useful to observe this alternating action of the mind with reference to heterogeneousness (increase of variety) and to coherence (unification). An idea is a *unit* though it may be complex, and is truth which is not presented by any of its parts. In the same way, our body is a unit which is something operative in the world in a way not provided for by any of its parts. This principle of the alternation of death and life in the mind was well observed by the ancient thinkers of India—mostly those Brahmins who in the social order were set apart from the struggle and the business of life, mainly, it seems, for the purpose of gaining, storing and handing on knowledge. They had a theory or doctrine of *maya,* which was their word for the method of creation of forms. The word has been translated "illusion" by many writers, because as it happens the same word is used to describe what in England and America we call conjuring shows. In India such shows are often given at street corners, round an itinerant showman and called *"mayas."* What these shows have in common with the natural creation of forms in the world and the mental creation of ideas in our minds is that in both cases something is hidden and something is displayed. It is on this account that interpreters have attached the idea of illusion to the formation of the created world. It is illusion only in the sense that we are seeing only a part of anything. We are seeing it in its separateness, not in its place in the whole. In science the illusion is accepted and called relativity, such that up is not up and down is not down—not really, only relatively.

There has been a lot of error in the understanding and interpretation of the idea of *maya*. Let us examine it carefully. *Maya* as creation or production of forms proceeds by two successive operations, called veiling and expressing. "Covering up" and "throwing forth" could also be suitable expressions to indicate the two successive operations involved in the production of a new form.

The first of these operations is a selection or limitation of materials—a putting of some of them out of sight or out of consideration. It is "operation exclusion," or "operation absence," that is to say, veiling, covering up, hiding, leaving out some things or something. Every time we decide to study or think about something we turn our whole attention to that and away from other things, that is we exclude as well as include—first exclude (concentration), then attend to what is included (study) and then observe its relations with other things (expansion). This study can be with the eyes open (examination), and even with the aid of various senses and actions (experimentation), but is still a concentration of attention upon a selected and limited field. When we have finished our thinking (study and expansion) we proceed to creative action, or else drop the matter and turn to something else. All this is an essential part of the old psychology of India. No doubt I have mentioned it before in these pages, but I want now to show its place in the creative process.

Now let us look at it in the old theory of creation of the universe. Creation in the Sanskrit language implies action *(kriya* or, in our modern spelling, *crea,* means something made), and this world of ours is frequently called, "the world of action" because in it forms are constantly being made and unmade. The act of creation is then described as taking place in two stages: the first by a word which means veiling, and the second by a word which means projecting.

To assure Sanskrit scholars that this is correct (others may skip this paragraph) I will give the words. The word which I have translated as veiling is *avarana* which is commonly used in poetry, drama, story-telling, etc., to mean covering or hiding; also sometimes with reference to a garment or other covering, to a shield, or even to a wall. For example, in the Raghuvansha there is a passage: *avaranaya drishteh kalpeta lokasya katham tamisra,* which I translate very literally as "How is the dark night qualified for hiding of the world from view?" In brief, Brahma, the Creator, when about to create the world, selected something and left something out. Really, there were two divinities engaged in this operation, Brahma and Vishnu; the former brought forward the material side of things, and the latter brought in the mind or life. They did these two jobs at the bidding of the originator of the whole business, Mahadeva. Strictly, these three were one being operating in three ways, just as a man may decide (will) to play golf, get himself clubs, etc. (thought and work), and then enjoy knocking the ball, etc. (feeling or emotion).

The idea here presented, if looked at scientifically, as an analysis of what we now actually find in our world of experience, would be that there are two kinds of being—one of materiality, the other of life. These are, so to speak, very tenacious, so that when the mind has made a form, that form is taken over by the material power and is now an object in the world.

Let me try to explain this projection more concretely. Suppose we are about to produce an automobile. Very well, then, we will leave out or reject certain things—swords, carpets, skillets, wastepaper baskets, geography books, etc. We are "covering up" or hiding part of the world which is within or around us and giving our attention to certain items exclusively. We are concentrating on something, and now we are looking at the not-rejected things —wheels, rods, cylinders, pipes, etc.—together. We are studying them closely, their characteristics. We are putting them together and fitting them together so that they are co-operating or coherent. If we are successful we have launched a new thing in the world. And there it is. We have thrown it out. So creation involves the two processes of rejecting and combining. Even in Genesis it is said that God created the heavens and the earth. Then, leaving the heavens aside, he proceeded to co-ordinate the "earth" into specific forms—molding the clay, as it were. Then he breathed the breath of life *(nephesh)* into Adam.

Such is the process called *maya,* and it is illusion to the extent that anything is not seen truly as it is, because it is not seen as a kind of eddy in the stream of things, nor in relation to all things, but is seen as an independent entity, and so the world looks like a collection of things, instead of a lot of nodes or balances in a continuous flow—not even then an interplay of somethings. In this flow materiality is required to account for space or extensity, and mind is required to account for time. However, that is somewhat beside our present theme, which is the inadequacy of the mind to relieve us of all pains, for the simple reason that it has great limitations, and has pains of its own. It is pertinent to our task to ask whether it can put us in harmony with the world so that we feel no antagonism to it or any of its parts or works, and the answer to that is "Yes it can assure us that the world is our friend." Or, in religious terms, it can assure us that "The Father knoweth of what ye have need," and "Not a sparrow falls to the ground without the Father." And, in our present view, we can include all the pains that exist as being in the prescription for our welfare, since work and achievement are necessary to the overcoming which will bring us to the fruit of the tree of true life.

There is another rather interesting theory from the East, which is becoming popular in the Western world at present, entitled Zen, a Japanese word meaning meditation, derived indirectly from the Sanskrit word *dhyana,* which means meditation, or as Patanjali describes it, a continued mental effort upon an object of concentration.[13]

This Far Eastern method of meditation, which was developed in
[13]*Yoga Sutras,* iii 1, 2.

China, to some extent from the old Tao school of thought of Lao-Tse and to some extent from the teaching of an Indian Buddhist missionary to China named Bodhidharma, follows the tendency of the Chinese mind in the direction of imagination (in the best sense, as the ability to receive and view pictures of real things in the mind), rather than the inferential or reasoning tendencies of the Hindu. The argument with the Zenists was not that a certain mode of thought would remove pain, but that a certain way of looking at things without thought would give great happiness, at least great serenity. From their point of view this was a matter of actual experience, but from ours, or at least mine, it would be because everything in nature gives us of its attainment if it is accepted as it is. You and I will no doubt feel more relaxed every time that we see a cat enjoying the luxury of its wonderful relaxation. A lady in one of my classes just could not sit up straight. Without telling her why, I asked her to meditate upon a tall stand lamp which had a beautiful straight pole about two and a half inches thick. After a while I saw her straighten up. This was a regular part of Patanjali's teaching. He would set his students to contemplate various natural objects not to *imitate* but to *appreciate* them.

Well, the point of Zen is that at all times, as far as possible, one should see things as they are and see them whole in this way. The formula for it is "no mind." If you are looking at a color you see it in this way, or, if you are hearing a sound. There is no *adhyasa* or mental bias, as a Vedantist would put it. Of course, this practice can be undertaken as a special exercise of this kind of meditation, but that would be necessary only for getting a true alignment and outlook. At the back is this trueness to nature. One sees the influence of this in Chinese paintings, and one finds it also to some extent in modern painting in which, not often enough, the artist is not trying to be clever. It must be said that some moderns have interpreted the idea of trusting to nature to include the idea of letting yourself go into impulsive pleasures which are by no means natural, forgetting that man himself is perhaps the one creature in nature who is not a fit subject for Zen contemplation. Certainly one's own self-image comes within that category.

I hope it has been shown in this chapter that it would be a great mistake to diminish the sense of self or I, and the greatest wisdom to give up, progressively, the wrong "self-image," "personality picture" or "mistaken identity."

When the Hindu speaks of liberation, it is liberation from these errors that is indicated. Although he believes that when the man has realized his true self he has finished his schooling and has no need of further incarnations in this limited condition of life, he also calls such a man a *jivanmukta,* that is, one who is liberated while still in embodied life.

Similarly, when Buddha spoke of nirvana, which means a blowing-out, as of a candle, the reference is to the blowing-out of the error of mistaken self-identity with its emotional attachments and their consequent actions and karmic effects.

I hope it has also been indicated that in the list of the five sources of trouble given early in this chapter two of them, desire and aversion, form a pair, so when there is a recommendation to "give up desire," it has to include "give up aversion." This will leave pleasures during the living, while the process of giving up erroneous self-images is going on, but those pleasures will no longer be "my pleasures," but body-pleasures, emotion-pleasures and mind-pleasures—in other words, pleasures of the animal in which I am at present residing. So, painful and unnatural austerities are out of place on the Path, and were denounced by Buddha and also by Krishna, the teacher of the *Bhagavad Gita.* Very important and helpful it is to know that our faults or deficiencies are temporary and are being corrected all the time, while our virtues or strengths are permanent. There is also the fact that our faults are not our own, but our virtues are.

Chapter 9

The Pains of Love

In the pursuit and discovery of knowledge there is a gain in power and facility of mind, which afterwards becomes available in the employment of the mind in practical affairs or in further enquiry and study. This statement might seem to show each individual as set in a state of isolation from all others so that he should do all his own finding out and all his own planning. But it contains its own antidote. Yes, each one of us is a separate being, advancing every day in the powers of will, love and thought by the use of these faculties, but the objects on which these faculties sharpen their teeth are of two kinds—material things and other living beings. The knowledge we seek may be not direct knowledge about iron or electricity, but other people's knowledge of these things. We find that two heads are better than one, just as two pairs of arms are better than one pair.

Our environment consists of not only things but also people, and even then not only the people as things (animate things), but as minds—and indeed it may be said that these numerous and varied minds, with their opinions and feelings and decisions to act, constitute the most important part of our world of information and experience. It is for this reason that it has been suggested that in the relations between individual and community it should be the chief solicitude of government to facilitate and encourage the individual in his own special capacities, and the chief solicitude of the individual to use his abilities in every transaction with others as much for the welfare of others as for himself. Thus comes to be known the collective value of love.

In course of development or evolution this social love comes to be a natural impulse and enjoyment, guiding the intellect of all the participants to larger and fuller growth.

Yet all these people—even the few or the one we love most—are outside us and it is one of the greatest pains of love that we can never get right into the beloved. We can know the thoughts, feelings and the desires to some extent—to a considerable extent sometimes — but try as we may we cannot put ourselves in his place and know and feel just what life is to him.

Is this another terrible pessimism?—that even love cannot release us from pain, but on the contrary has a form of pain built into it in the shape of this impossibility of complete fulfilment, and this built-in hunger for that impossible.

Not so, but quite the reverse, if we apply the analogy so far proven valid, that in the maturing of each capacity in turn, there is the formation of the seedbed for the birth of the next. In this manner, hunger broke through and gave rise to emotions, emotions led to larger life but also many troubles. These troubles could not be solved by emotion, so mental intelligence came in to solve them. But mental intelligence became embittered by its own kind of greed—first intelligence in service of emotional desires, and then intelligence with its own greed for knowledge, and then the same kind of thing *ad infinitum,* and, what is worse, the discovery that all its items have only a relative validity, and there is no knowledge of the essential ingredients of its increasing edifice of knowledge. This frustration was solved by the birth of love; that which, piercing the individual's mental egotism as from above, informs the individual in a new way, so that he cares in his very heart what happens to another. The welfare of another or others becomes to him as vital as his own—becomes vital *like* his own, since without his own he could not realize theirs.

The maturity of this love comes when it triumphs over the thinking mind, and that mind realizes that this alone can give it satisfactory motive and direction. Then another achievement comes when that mind looks at human politics and history (individual and collective) and sees that where love has been used it has justified its existence. The intellect does not cease its working—the man has not become a fool—but it sees that what Emerson called "divine arithmetic" is a fact, that when individual joins individual in the pursuit of prosperity or knowledge (with true love, "on the square" and "on the level") one and one do not make two, but perhaps twenty or two hundred. This is the lesson of love in family, in friendship, in labor and in society.

This is surely the lesson for present-day humanity. The logical faculty is now mature in practically all people. Nothing can improve its function and structure, any more than it can convert our legs into wheels or our arms into cranes and bull-dozers. But this vast new and transforming lesson of love is being learnt by the bitter method of pain—and yet to some extent by wisdom, the realization that love is greater than thought. Indeed, thought is richer for its coming, and desire is richer, and material living is richer, all of them in both quality and power.

Love is the present lesson of mankind—especially that which has been called "love of neighbor," for this is no cloud-land but applies with all the individual's specific relation to that portion of the world with which he is in touch—where his power to act lies, and where his knowledge applies. It may be recalled that when Jesus was asked, regarding his advice to love our neighbor, what the word neighbor signified, he cited the case of the good Samaritan, who found a man hurt by the roadside and took care of him. The word neighbor means "someone who is nigh," some one or more with whom we are in touch. As I am quoting Jesus, let us remember also the statement: "None cometh to the Father but through me"—speaking as the conscious embodiment of love, spoken of in another place as the living bread which cometh down from heaven, so that he who feeds his life with that will come to experience the life immortal. It may be recalled also that he set all his followers a task—they must love! This was not to be done for them; it was their task.

That this wonderful love should have its pains, even when it is most ascendant, is no cause for sadness either. It can be taken as the seedbed for the next newness of realization of what life is. We have seen that life is taking and giving, with joy of senses and limbs; that it is also feeling; that it is also thinking; and now it is also loving, and still further, though we may see yet only dimly, we do see that a new light is breaking through which can assure the mind that not only truth and love are justified in fact, but these justifications warrant also the opinion that the present unity of interest and welfare which love presents will be followed by some conscious realization of the unity of our very life. In the triumvirate of universal relationships, as Unity, Harmony and Variety, we can see love as harmony, but unity is still a mystery, though a fact.

"What then! Are you going against that very individuality which has made even love possible? Such would seem to be the case in a doctrine or theory of unity!"

No, sirs. No indeed. Such an idea would be a shocking anthropomorphism. One cannot describe feelings in terms of material forms, nor intellect in terms of feeling, nor love in terms of intellect—nor this, which we are thinking *of,* not thinking *about*—even in terms of love. Perhaps the term "transcendental" may be used, if it is remembered that nothing is omitted but everything is seen in a new light, in which the reality is that everything is seen in unity.

I have a small simile or analogy for this. Picture a sculptor talking in his studio to a friend, promising him a statue from a block of marble which is there. "What would you like," he asks, "a child's head, an animal, a bird, a pagoda?" The friend puzzles for a while and then says, "A bird." A few days later the bird is ready; the sculptor has chipped away the unwanted pieces of stone, and has left the bird—yes, not made the bird, but *left* the bird form which was already there. I reflect that the child's head, the pagoda and many other things were also there in that block of marble and if the friend had asked for a pagoda, then likewise the unwanted portion would have been chipped away and the wanted portion left. Those forms are all there but in unity, in reality.

It may be a play upon words, but I reflect that reality means royalty, and royalty is what is above the law, above restrictions, somewhat as Patanjali dared to offer a definition of God as—to put the idea in modern words—that being who has no subjection to anything other. A similar idea was presented by another ancient writer, who believed that the act of creation was a "spreading-out" of all this, in space and time, in terms of here and there and of then and now. Again the creation was declared to be produced by thought—by a mental act, which begins with a limitation, just as our sculptor so began his piece of work. This we see in fact, as bearing on the reality and power of unity, that not one piece or parcel of anything, whether of matter or of mind, can get away from this universe and have an existence separately, by itself.

It may interest some readers of these pages who have been studying religious ideas coming from various ancient nations, to know that this very same thought is behind the constant recital of the word Om by Hindu devotees. The letter o is a compound vowel or diphthong, beginning with the sound of a (as in pat), and gliding instantly into u (as in put). This is, so to say, the beginning and the middle of the word Om (sounded like home without the h). The a is a throat sound, from the very back of the mouth, the first or beginning sound of our human utterance, and the m sound is the last of such sounds, made with the lips closed. So the word Om is considered to be the epitome and container of all human words, and therefore the correct word with which to indicate our idea of God. So, again Patanjali writes that when Om is recited it should be done with intentness upon its meaning. We may note that it is not descriptive.

So also we find it in the famous *Bhagavad Gita,* scripture of the intellectuals of old India. There it is said that aspirants to the wiser life begin all their undertakings with the recital, *"Om tat sat,"* which means "Om—that is the reality." So, whatever may be the object in view in any piece of work, it is remembered that it is not in itself important, except as a step on the way to that reality or realization.

Is the same truth also indicated in Hymn 65 given in *Hymns of the Spirit* (published by the Beacon Press, Inc., Boston, Mass.) as follows?

> Thou whose spirit dwells in all,
> Primal source of life and mind,
> In the clod as in the soul,
> Ever full and unconfined!
>
> What shall separate from thee?
> Naught of all created things!
> Joy and sorrow, good and ill,
> Each from thee its essence brings.

I have often thought that if the statement of Jesus regarding sparrows, that even "One of them shall not fall on the ground without your Father" is accurately represented, he was speaking of the doctrine of the absolute presence, not referring to a being in any sense away or apart. This, because it is not "without your Father's knowledge of it," but "without your Father." The Father is indicated not as any sort of thing, or energy, or person, or mind, but as of the nature of that ubiquitous power which is by some religious philosophers called Law. This is not an abstraction. It is more, not less. The sparrow is that, too, but wearing many veils.

It will be noticed that law differs from force and matter in that it is not *in the stream* of events, and is in no way expendable, as they are, but appears "out of the blue" when its working is appropriate. It is truly beyond space and time.

Chapter 10

Beyond the Stoics

In Chapter 7 we have observed the outlook of the Stoic and seen to what splendid self-reliance and peace of mind it leads—peace in the sense of adequacy to all occasions, not in the sense of passivity or resignation. Let us now see how with our modern sense of law in nature this self-reliant outlook can be blended with progress on the one hand and gratitude for the gift and joy of life on the other.

In that chapter we compared the Stoic with the Epicurean. Let us now compare him with the Platonist, so that all three may be combined. It is grand for any of us to have studied the value of the Epicurean life, and the Stoic life, and the Platonic life, separately. Those three "concentrations" will have revealed to us their merits, but now, in our day, with the conception of Law over all, we can see the combination, or rather the unity of the three.

Let us proceed, then, to comparison, the "meditation" part of this theme. The Stoic was a man of will, who decided that life ought to be lived according to the decisions of the mind, and that there could be no greater mistake than that of allowing things to drift "according to nature." It has long been observed that everything that is left to the course of nature decays and perishes. Only those objects or structures that are favored with the possession of an indwelling mind or at least an instinct of self-preservation, exhibit growth and progress; and even the living body itself decays—every act of life is an operation of decay or partial death—and has to be restored to strength by an indwelling instinct that arranges for its nourishment and protection. A wise man carefully trains his dogs and horses, stands guard over the health of his own body and constantly repairs and restores his land and houses. The mind is the source of creative activity. Matter left to itself produces no organic structures at all.

So this mind is the most precious thing, and man does need to regulate his personal life by its arts, and to exercise its faculties by use in all the affairs of life. Let man, then, stand firmly on this pedestal, and from his own mind determine the course and the details of his life, and not trouble himself with that which lies outside his power.

Perhaps the greatest deterrent to the clear and full use of this faculty is agitation, the result of fear, regret, anxiety. On this account it became a cardinal act of faith with the Stoics to concern the mind only with those things that seemed to lie within its power, to such an extent that almost the first thing a Stoic would do when confronted with anything that seemed to call for his thought or action would be to put to himself the question, "Is this a matter within my power or not?" And if it were not, he would dismiss it from his mind and not permit himself to be troubled about it.

But there was one thing that he did most heartily fear—that in the region of things within his power he might fail to use his faculties to the best of his power. The Stoic carried this philosophical detachment to such a degree that when a man was thrown into prison he would not trouble himself about it, but would say to his jailors, "You have taken possession of that body that I used to call mine, and the responsibility for its welfare now devolves upon you; I shall not trouble my mind about it." And the man would always regulate his affairs so that he would not become a slave to any material possessions; if he did not feel great enough in character to manage them without anxiety he would let them go and take to a simpler life.

The Platonists, however, found this doctrine insufficient. They felt it necessary to examine the status of the mind itself, and to seek the source from which it derived its strength. They put to themselves the question "What is this mind, and whence comes its power?" And in order to make a study of that they considered the nature of the best sort of mind—that of the genius.

Now, to the Greeks, there were two best sorts of genius—that of the philosopher and that of the artist—which bore fruit of truth and beauty, respectively. Then the question arose, "Does the philosopher make with his mind the truth he sees, or does he *discover* it in the entire world?" Surely, he does not make it. "And is the great sculptor or artist an inventor or a copyist?" He is a copyist. But let us not mistake the greatness of his function. He is above other men, because he sees beauty where they are blind.

The argument continues: "If it takes the mind of the greatest genius among men merely to perceive and copy the original, what must be the nature of the genius by whom the original was brought into being?" Bow down, then, before that "Divine Mind" which pervades the whole universe. In it lies the source of our understanding, our love and our power. Reverence that, worship that, so that in the close contact with it that devotion gives we may imbibe its greatness and enjoy it in our own life.

In some there is an awakening here of something that is beyond even the perceptions of genius in the world. This contemplation leads to an experience of that which is above all dependency and therefore beyond loss. It is an experience within oneself and yet concerning also the world, and it carries with it its own incredible joy. May I say that it is an experience of the Original Power! That is the meaning of the word divine. It seems to derive from an old Sanskrit verbal root, *div,* which means to shine, and has led to many other words, such as "deity" and "day." This shining is the original light of all powers, as contrasted with reflected or dependent light—the sun, in old symbology, as contrasted with the moon. Does not this awakening account for the ecstasies of the artist and the philosopher, which are beyond all egoic expansions or enhancements? Something of this awakening could have accounted for Emerson's bold statement that "Worship is the flowering and completion of human culture."

We must not forget, of course, that the artist is a producer as well as a seer, that in his work there is skill as well as vision. He adds to his developed perception of the beauty that lies in the true nature of things the skill to reproduce it under conditions that draw the attention of other men to it. Thus the artist is a teacher. Art does not exist for its own sake, but for the education of men so that they may at last see for themselves the beauty that is everywhere. Probably this sort of education is within the experience of most of us. You may, for example, have gone to look over a gallery of paintings, and exclaimed, as many have done before a splendid picture of a sunset, "Why! Surely no such colors as these ever existed in the sky!" But the next time your eye fell upon a real sunset, you said with wonder, "There are the colors that the artist depicted on his canvas."

What is true in this as regards the artist is true also of the philosopher, who could be described as an artist in words, and he it seems is at his best when he is a poet. Why is it that a truth expressed in poetry is so much more effective than the same stated in prose? The answer is simple. The poetic form creates a pause and a poise. By being discontinuous it creates moments of pure contemplation of the stated truth. However short the moment may be it is revelatory, or at the very least concentrational, for the vision does not "take time." The work of the artist also creates a concentration or a contemplation upon the truth of beauty that he presents. If it is a statue he puts it on a pedestal; if it is a picture he puts it in a frame, which also checks the wandering of the mind and causes a return to the proper theme of the artist's work. A bracelet on the wrist has something of the same function, as an aid to the perception of the beauty of the hand.

One of my favorite thoughts is that we all carry along with us a share of the Original Power. We feel it in our consciousness in that we credit ourselves with the sense that "I act" or "I do." Even when we are saying to ourselves, "I walk" there is the same cryptic assertion. Surprisingly to those who have not yet thought of it this sharing of original power can be shown to be true even of the body, as, for example, when it walks. The argument from gravitation proclaims this element of independence in the body, for just as apples do not fall to the ground, but the apple and the ground both positively attract each other and move accordingly, so it can be said that when we stand up the earth not only supports the body, but the body also supports the earth, though in the lesser measure of its smaller mass.

In a more abstract statement, if five bodies, say stars, form a group or unit, influencing one another by their masses, momentums and orbits, and we call them A, B, C, D, and E, then if A is influenced by B to E, it is still not totally influenced. A can also be shown to be an influencer with respect to the dependency of B, C, D or E. Therefore also A is one of the influencers of itself when A is influenced by B, C, D and E. In brief, each one of them has a portion or a share of the original power and independence. Therefore also it is true that when we walk we float or fly—what *is* the proper word?—in some degree. I have no doubt that this is the secret of the will. It is also perhaps the secret of such truths as, "A thing of beauty is a joy forever" and "Art alone endures."

The faith in natural law which sustains the modern scientist in his researches and in the applications of his science to material industry is also, if straightly viewed, a similar sort of worship. If the scientist allows himself to feel about this, as well as to think about it—which is not often the case—he will find himself full of gratitude that he is in a world of law or cosmos and not of chaos, and perhaps also of wide-eyed wonder that this can be so, in a world in which everything he sees has no authenticity of its own. This gratitude and wonder is very much akin to the worship of the devotee.

The scientific man, like the artist and the philosopher, is also two-sided. He has skills as well as vision. A very modern aspect of this matter is to be seen in the achievements of scientific genius. With faith in the world and devotion to truth, the men of science have allied mankind with unseen and wonderful powers of nature, and thereby enriched our lives enormously. There are no greater devotees than these, who have perfect faith in the rational or intelligible order of the world, yet more valuable by far than any material profit is the enrichment that they have brought to the growing mind of man, giving out a larger view, a stronger foundation of self-confidence, and enhancement of power. Their work clearly exhibits the possibilities of man's achievement when self-reliance and devotion blend in one attitude of mind.

One of the most illuminating ideas in Hindu scripture is that relating to the creation of the solar system. In that legend, when God the Father (Shiva) told the Holy Spirit (Brahma) to form the universe, what did he do? He sat down in meditation and as he thought the forms of matter came into being. Thought is the activity of the mind; motion is the activity of matter. Herein lies the secret of our present immortality, for those who care to meditate upon it. And just as in the material world we ally our bodily powers with the forces of steam and electricity in order to share in a life larger than that which this little body can provide, so, surrendering ourselves with the science of the soul to the uses of the divine thought and love and power that permeate the world, we become part of a richer consciousness than what we formerly thought to be our own. Such is the Platonist ideal.

This kind of devotion is the inspiration of a creation *through* man himself of his own perfection with the aid of all the world. The future may be reasoned to be as much above the status of present-day civilized man as he is above the most primitive man of whom we have any knowledge. This kind of *devotion* is evolutionally far beyond earlier man's *obedience,* for with this outlook he is on his feet, with no doors closed before him, with no chains upon his will, love and thought. Julian Huxley has given us a very apposite thought in this matter: "If the religious believe that the spirit of truth be a gift from or a part of the third person of the Trinity, then to continue to shut oneself up in the swaddling-clothes of primitive doctrine when the limbs of the spirit might be freed for action, is a sin against the Holy Ghost."[14]

It is interesting that Jesus called himself "Son of Man" as well as "Son of God," indicating that the perfect man is self-made though not alone. And he said, too, that "Your Father knoweth of what you have need"—at all times, everywhere—which should put all the gods and gurus and priests, insofar as they try to govern others on the road to the goal of life, entirely out of business; just as Buddha did when he taught self-confidence and trust in the Good Law.

[14] *Religion Without Revelation,* by Julian Huxley, p. 175, (Mentor Series).

>..Seek
> Nought from the helpless gods by gift and hymn,
>   Nor bribe with blood, nor feed with fruit and cakes;
> Within yourselves deliverance must be sought;
>   Each man his prison makes.

And:

> Such is the Law which moves to righteousness,
>   Which none at last can turn aside or stay;
> The heart of it is Love, the end of it
>   Is Peace and Consummation sweet. Obey![15]

It was never suggested that reason is greater than love. The Law was of the nature of love as well as of reason. Buddha was as insistent as Jesus upon the law and life of love being the law for man, as may be seen in his list of the "noble eightfold path." It is true that Buddha identified the Good Law with the law of karma, the doctrine that man not only will reap as he sows, but is now reaping as he has sown in the past. It is true also that he held that the future reaping would take place in this world of rational life and educative experience. I think, too, that Jesus must have had the same idea in mind when he said: "Judge not, and ye shall not be judged: condemn not, and ye shall not be condemned: forgive, and ye shall be forgiven: Give, and it shall be given unto you; good measure, pressed down, and shaken together, and running over, shall *men* give into your bosom. For with the same measure that ye mete withall it shall be measured to you again."[16] I have italicized the word *men* in this passage. If all the unrequited good in the world is to be repaid *by men,* I think the doers thereof must come back into this world in new incarnations to receive it.

Buddha's point was that:

> More is the treasure of the Law than gems;
>   Sweeter than comb its sweetness; its delights
> Delightful past compare.

. . . .

[15]*The Light of Asia,* by Sir Edwin Arnold.
[16]Luke 6: 38.

>   . . . . .Utter true
>   Its measures mete, its faultless balance weighs;
>   Times are as nought, tomorrow it will judge
>   Or after many days.[17]

and yet it was, as we quoted, "the law that moves to righteousness"—educative not punitive.

And above all it is to be noted that this law is educative to love, not merely educative to what to do and what not to do. I see in this the answer to a great sadness expressed by a distinguished modern writer and student of human nature, W. Somerset Maugham. In one place he says:

> "But I have seen a child die of meningitis. I have only found one explanation that appealed equally to my sensibility and to my imagination. This is the doctrine of the transmigration of souls. As everyone knows, it assumes that life does not begin at birth or end at death, but is a link in an indefinite series of lives . . . each one of which is determined by the acts done in previous existences . . . It would be less difficult to bear the evils of one's own life if one could think that they were but the necessary outcome of one's errors in a previous existence, and the effort to do better would be less difficult too when there was the hope that in another existence a greater happiness would reward one. But if one feels one's own woes in a more forcible way than those of others it is the woes of others that arouse one's own indignation. It is possible to achieve resignation in regard to one's own, but only philosophers obsessed with the perfection of the Absolute can look upon those of others, which seem so often unmerited, with an equal mind. If karma were true one could look upon them with pity, but fortitude. Revulsion would be out of place and life would be robbed of the meaninglessness of pain which is pessimism's unanswered argument. I can only regret that I find the doctrine as impossible to believe as the solipsism of which I spoke just now."[18]

[17] *The Light of Asia,* by Sir Edwin Arnold.
[18] *Mr. Maugham Himself,* p. 656. Doubleday & Co., New York.

The answer to Mr. Maugham's difficulty is that material troubles are to be regarded as brought to us by the law of karma, but the education it brings to man includes the education to love and of love. We are to develop love for all, and then to face the pains of love. Rationally, these pains should not be diminished by reason; rather love will learn through sympathy to develop not fortitude but sensitiveness, and the impulse to act more according to love in future by having more love where the love was deficient before.

Sympathy is the awakener of love; love is the father and mother of good deeds, and good deeds alone will bring material suffering to an end. When there is not love there are hurtful deeds, and hurtful deeds are the offspring of action without understanding love. The karma doctrine is not for escape or consolation, but for teaching us to co-operate willingly, heartily and intelligently in the process of awakening—education, which means "leading out."

I notice that in a modern novel there is a passage which agrees with this idea that criminal acts are due to deficiency of love. One of the characters, a personality analyst, speaking about a criminal family, says: "The thing that made these people what they were wasn't a positive quality, but a negative one. It was a lack of something in them from the beginning, not something they'd acquired."[19]

In a book *Character Building* which I wrote in 1923, I showed in detail how harmful acts arose out of deficiencies of character. Taking laziness, thoughtlessness and selfishness, as the three cardinal sins of character, it was easy to point out that strength in one or two of the three qualities of will, love and thought with deficiency in another of them was the chief cause of human trouble. For example, a strong will and a powerful intellect with love deficiency, or a strong and great love with an intellect deficiency, or a great love with a will deficiency. In this it will be noticed that the will is not to be defined as the strongest or prevailing emotion, as some do, but as a self-control which gives decision and a persistency to live and act in the face of difficulties. Weakness in all three directions would never lead to strong acts, such as could

[19]*The Bad Seed,* by Richard Marsh.

have conspicuous effects in the field of karma. It is also argued that few people can be trusted with great power, because of this unbalance of the three characteristics.

When we come to the question as to why there is *so much* karmic suffering in the world—we have only to look in the pages of our social and political history books to see plenty of cause. One of the worst has been religious fanaticism, including terrible deeds done even in the name of love. The ways in which people have hurt one another are uncountable, the degree and volume of their insensitive selfishness in some cases and their unintelligent love in others. The law of karma, striking at these, helps by arousing sensitiveness and thus is the complete two-fold inner and outer law of benefit to every living being. It is to be noticed that if this theory of deficiency be true, as it seems to be, men have no faults, have nothing to lose or shred off, but only the necessity to grow in love, or in thought, or in will, as the case may be.

Such is the law of karma, as it is briefly called, which has been expounded widely and with great labor and assiduity throughout the Western world by the members of The Theosophical Society in much the same terms as it has been told for thousands of years by the Buddhists and Hindus in the East. For this service a great number of people have had reason to be profoundly grateful to the numerous nameless students and workers of that Society.

Speaking of myself, I contacted this doctrine back in the 1890's in the pages of Sir Edwin Arnold's book, about two years before I knew about The Theosophical Society. I at once felt that it was the only doctrine that could explain how it was that man had "risen so much higher than his source" and could also give a reason for what has been called his "divine discontent." By its emphasis on "the good law" it added to the rational picture of the world—just the one thing needed by a young scientist to enable him to add to his feeling of deep gratitude to the world for its rational or non-chaotic character, a further gratitude for its opening the door to every man to the achievement of a goal which all men want, but from which in the West they are all around falling back frustrated because they think the school or the arena will soon be closed to them by death. In this view there was also release of heart, mind and will from the bondage of chance or caprice.

I was already acquainted with the work of the scientific spiritualists, as two of my uncles were deeply interested in that research, but I could not see that progress after death in a world not containing our present difficulties and limitations could lead to mental and moral growth, nor justify the existence of a world like this full of trouble if it were not useful and necessary. This world of ours is both useful and necessary, and we see in it people at different stages of growth, so we may consider it reasonable to think that reincarnation is the most probable mode. It is no use saying that we should wait until we know. The way of life is to act upon our best judgment. Indeed it has been remarked that even if people do not believe themselves immortal they had better act as if they did in order to make a success of their mortal life, and find a reason to remain in harness to the end and die on their feet.

But why should a karmic effect be experienced at a particular time and place? Because it flows in, as it were, when the vacuum occurs. Like other laws, it operates when the opportunity arises. It is pending all the time, or, on the analogy of physical forces, is "potential," until an occasion for discharge occurs. This refers to what the old books call karma in storage *(sanchita karma),* but all agree that the vast bulk of our karma is of the ready-money kind *(kriyamana karma),* as when we overeat and have indigestion, or as a riotous youth leads to decrepit age. Third and last in this classification of karmic effects is that which is currently occurring *(prarabha karma),* which include our condition of birth, with a certain kind of body and environment, and whatever from the storage may have discharged itself upon us at a given time. Along with all this is the further statement that all good now being freely done cancels out old cruelties and unkindnesses still in our storage, so that they may never come, besides providing us with an extended field of education.

All this comes within the law of causality: "The same combination always produces the same effect." It is law; and all law, including natural law, can always be relied upon. That is what makes the world understandable, so that, philosophically speaking, we live in an intelligible world—a cosmos, not a chaos. There is nothing more reliable, so to say, than the material world. If the stars came down to dance on the village green on Monday, and went for a cruise of the Pacific Ocean on Tuesday, and all things so erratically acted, our minds could not plan at all, could not even think. The existence of such minds as ours in the world implies this orderliness in nature, and the corollary is that mind should always seek to know the laws of nature and life and work with them.

In man there is obviously a mind element in every cause and effect—a thought, an emotion, or a decision. Without that feature called mind in the stream of causation there would not be a clock or an ocean liner in the world. This mind is definitely responsible for certains forms in the world, not only clocks and steamboats, but also the form of the human body to a large extent. Even the formation of the bodies of the birds and squirrels can be traced back to that hunger of life which is seen as actions and emotions leading to modifications of form to suit the environment.

The logical minds of the intellectuals of old India also led them to this understanding and appreciation of law. This is attested by their old books of science *(Sankhya* and *Vaisheshika)* and logic *(Nyaya)*. They went further and said in effect, "If the orderliness in nature goes along with intellect in man, so also there must be a good law in nature corresponding to the goodness in man—a law which nurtures that goodness." The rising of the thought-mind in man is paralleled by the rising of the love-mind. As thought grows and rejoices in the world because of truth in the world, so love grows and rejoices in the world because of a natural good law.

Thus appear the two laws—the inner law of life which is the method of growth by use and exercise, and the outer law of karma which is the method of rewarding will, love and thought and correcting the deficiencies. The two together are sufficient to guarantee evolution, provided that life goes on. Both laws provide for sensitiveness to the consciousness in others (love), and for sensible and effective dealing with things and situations (thought and will). Some have remarked that in the theory of karma, the law takes care of "sins of omission" as well as of commission, but in fact all sins seem to be sins of omission—omission of will, love, or thought in some respect. Still, it is the law of action, for karma means action, or, more accurately doing, or, still more accurately, making. In this world what you make you have, and it stands until it is unmade.

Chapter 11

Knowledge, Law and Life

All of us who have a scientific bent have considerable liking for probability. We value it for two reasons—one is that we are not absolutely sure of anything in this world, since our basic ideas about matter and other things have let us down so badly in the comparatively recent past, and logically, we are dependent upon syllogistic reasoning with its defective premises. The other reason is—as Dr. Harry Emerson Fosdick so aptly remarked on one occasion—even if you cannot make up your mind you have to make up your life.

We must act, and must do so on the basis of the highest probability. This means that our lives must be to some extent experimental; we are still subject to the method of trial and error, like our little friend the paramecium. But we have made a great advance beyond the status of that little animal. We have in our minds thousands of memories of past experiences which give us inner guidance as to the best angle through which to turn on a given occasion, when we wish either to try something new, or having tried and missed, to try again.

Not only have we available in our minds this great collection of memories, we have also the ability to reason out a probability to guide our action in cases in which we have had no previous experience. This thinking-box gives us a great advantage. Instead of blundering forward, backing off, changing our angle and trying again—the method of trial and error—we can do more or less thinking about the situation before we act, come to a conclusion about the highest probability with reference to what we desire, and then, after decision, try again. If the idea on which we have acted pays off, we say that it must be correct and must represent some truth or reality around us. We speak of it as verified by experience. All the same, we cannot be completely sure even that the sun will rise tomorrow; we can only have an extremely high expectation of it—not a hundred per cent certainty.

Now, with regard to the idea of karma. It is of the nature of law which, as in the case of truth, does not need to travel or transit in order to be operative. If angels or gods there be, they must be of this nature and operation, not of the nature of mind or matter, but of unlimited life. Let us do Buddha justice in remembering that he said he *knew,* and that to him karma as law definitely was a fact in nature. It is very significant that Buddha had such a modern point of view that he did not credit the operations of nature to the planning or functioning of any God or gods, but called the law of karma simply a law. Although he taught the idea of nirvana as the ending of the series of births or bodies, to be attained by each individual as he overcomes the weaknesses which keep him under the dominion of the law of karma, he maintained that it is a condition of happiness, and a state superior to that of any God or gods which men have pictured. None of the qualities of either mind or body could be attributed to that state, because all such qualities are nothing but limitations or defects, although they seem to ignorant men to be powers and delights.

Some people—many millions, and even now it is estimated that there are more Buddhists in the world than people of any other creed—have "followed" Buddha, because of their confidence in his leadership, which appeals to both their reason and brotherhood feelings. The modern Theosophists, while differing in their views of minor matters, all agree, I believe, in the ideas of reincarnation and karma, and all say, I believe, that if anyone propounds a religious idea which violates reason or love, such an idea is to be rejected outright. These Theosophists number approximately thirty-five thousand in the western hemisphere, officially entered on the books of the Society, and there is a penumbra of uncommitted sympathizers amounting to perhaps ten times that number, so that the Society and movement represent a considerable body of free thought and conviction on these subjects.

Although following their leader, as the Buddhists do, rests upon a belief in the reliability of Buddha's thinking or illumination in this matter, the Buddhists will tell you that they have not surrendered their independence of judgment and decision, and that their trust in their leader is based upon their reasoned opinion of him and his doctrine. Psychologically, we know, no man can get away from responsibility to himself, but there is such a thing as mass hypnosis to which he may choose to yield. The most that the *thinking* man can say is that the doctrine is in the *highest* degree probable. This would remain true even if one realized that Buddha did not know the law by means of his thinking mind, which always deals in probabilities, but by some superior means, which we may call direct perception. Incidentally, in the *Bhagavad Gita,* Krishna makes the same claim to the same kind of knowledge.

But now back to our principle of probability. First the scientific. We have already observed in an earlier chapter that evolution is taking place in nature. We see that this agrees very well with Herbert Spencer's classical definition of evolution already quoted: "A progressive change from a state of incoherent homogeneity to a state of coherent heterogeneity of structure and function." Incoherent means, of course, that the parts are not operating for mutual support and gain. In a tree, for example, the various branches are competing for the sunlight, but in an animal or in a man the various "branches," called arms, legs, eyes, ears, etc. are cohering. Further they are heterogeneous, that is variously specialized instead of being similar or homogeneous as are the branches of a tree.

The thinking capacity of a man provides an ability to appraise a combination of events—a complex occurrence—which has never before presented itself either in that man's experience or in that of his ancestors. Consider, for example, the complexity of a certain position of the chessmen on a chess-board in the middle of a game. It has been said that no two games of any reasonable length have ever been the same. There is in our lives constantly a newness to intrigue the mind and give it the pleasure of new activity, and enhancement of power, or the sense of dynamic being. This faculty of thinking has evolved and is evolving, not by the inclusion or gift of anything from outside it, but by the exercise of its own proper activity among things, just as is also the case with arms and legs. Indeed, we may safely say that it is the growth of this faculty of thinking which constitutes the main part of man's evolution at the present time. Arms and legs cease to grow about the age of, shall we say, twenty-one years, but the mind goes on growing as long as we live, if there is health.

Although the mind thus grows by studying, comparing, classifying and rearranging the things which surround it in the world, those things must not grow—they must continue to be just what they are. Their character must be "not-growth." If they were to grow or change the mind could not make use of them. In brief, while thought grows the objects of thinking do not. If the mountains were liable to dance about and leap into the sky, we certainly could not make useful maps of the countryside, or if in the town the businessmen's offices decided to play musical chairs with one another, carrying the men with them, we should be unable to think or plan our business.

The fact is that life, if thinking is life, needs death, if death is deadness, as its material for study, thinking and action. This world of deadness, or dead things is just as requisite for the play of life as life itself is. But someone says, "What of the plants and animals, and what of the seasons and of meteorological phenomena?"

The answer to this is that deadness does not preclude movement, but it is predictable movement. It is part of the deadness of water that it flows downhill. We can take that into our calculations, but could not do so if it flowed sometimes uphill and sometimes downhill, "without rhyme or reason," as we say, though we then speak very incongruously, as what we mean is without deadness.

All momentum is also part of the deadness. The billiard ball goes on rolling until friction or collision stops it. In the case of plants and animals, we must say that they are partly alive, just as we humans are partly alive, but not in the same degree. I cannot predict in what way the squirrel in the garden will jump and run when he sees me coming, but I will venture to believe that his view of me and his collection of memories, or rather recognitions, will have something to do with it. As explained before, he has not the memory and power of reason that man has, but he has only a "museum" mind.

Well, then, we have two classes of things set over against each other, those of death and those of life. These two are dancing together, like a man and a woman in a ballroom. In a human being the two are together as mind and body. It is not that the body is for most people a subject of study and experiment, an object of interest. It is a vehicle of sense-organs and of action, and has an intermediate function, so to say, between life and matter, whereby this life may study and experiment with the things of the world outside the body. From the standpoint of the life it is an instrument or tool, or a compendium of various instruments and tools.

The question for any one of us at any moment is: "Are you interested in more life or in more body?" After the body is full grown more body cannot mean more growth—but it could mean more health and strength if those are deficient. More body may also mean more possessions, security, comfort and pleasures of sensation. There is so much of this in human life that it is no wonder that St. Paul came out with the stern words: "Ye are dead, and your life is hid with Christ in God."

It is of great interest that though the animals are seen to have an "instinct of self-preservation," they must be credited also with an instinct to adventure. I recollect the statement of a scientific naturalist with relation to a squirrel he had been watching. This little animal, he said, was enticing a hawk to swoop down upon it. Every time that the hawk came down the squirrel would jump aside and hide behind a tree, and then, when the hawk was back up on a branch he would repeat the experiment apparently just for the enjoyment of the excitement of it. Patanjali added that advanced man has also an instinct to fulfilment *(apavarga)*.

The two things—the dead and the alive—are both obviously necessary to this business of living. One of them cannot be derived from the other. Much ingenuity has been expended by materialistic scientists in trying to show that life could have been derived from matter, or, in brief, that even our most complex and inclusive mentalizings are nothing more than highly complicated reflex actions. We are familiar with bodily reflexes, such as those which take place when sitting on a chair with one leg hanging over the knee of the other, and some one, perhaps the doctor, gives a little tap to the upper leg just below the knee, whereupon the leg gives a jump altogether out of proportion to the tap on it. There are many such reflexes in the body (also incidentally, in the lower mind), but these reflexes all take place without the accompaniment of consciousness. If then the active mind were merely a reflex even the most complicated thinking would be entirely unconscious; there would be no need of consciousness at all.

It is worth noticing that we know our bodies by observation of them, as with any other outward object. Toothache does not give us a mental picture of teeth and gums. It only says, "Something wrong here," and leaves it to us to find out what that something is. Further, we have to investigate and look at it *as an outside thing* to find that out. Without a mirror no would know what his face looks like. I remember occasions when travelling in Pullman cars and, waking up in the night, I could not tell which way my body was going—head first or feet first—until I let up the window blind, looked out at the occasional lights passing by, and from that inferred the direction of my own movement. We may travel in a jet plane at 600 miles an hour. It seems no different from slow travel, and indeed if we could have bodies made of whatever light or the light-wave is made of, we could, no doubt, travel 186,000 miles per second without knowing it. Anyhow, those of us who are living not far from the equator are revolving with the earth at the rate of about a thousand miles an hour, and along with the earth in its orbit we travel round the sun at about nineteen miles per second.

Even if life and matter are fundamentally one thing, that thing is not of the nature of matter. That basic "one thing" is not matter. You may say also it is not life either. Let us say, then, that life and matter are essentially one thing, but are that basic thing either subject to two different limitations, or expressing itself in two different ways. In this world, in either case, we find the two mingling, at least in human and animal forms.

Now some one may point out the fact that matter can be present without life. One scientist insisted upon explaining to me at length that he had a photographic camera with an automatic flashlight which went off in the dark at a fixed time and took a picture of what was there, in the entire absence of any person. Yes, that well illustrates the situation. But if matter and life are two different realities, not dependent upon each other for their essential nature and we find that material forms and even material actions can go on without life, we may not be unreasonable in assuming that life or mind can go on, and even the activity of life or mind can go on, without the presence of matter. In this view, just as material forms produced by mind can go on without that mind, so can the operations of the mind go on with the thoughts which have got into it as the result of its contact with matter, even if it is no longer in contact with that matter. And just as material forms can traffic with material forms in the absence of mind, so can mind traffic with mind in the absence of material forms. This fact has been conclusively demonstrated in what is called "thought-transference." I must not relate my own numerous experiences and experiments in this field—this book would grow too big—but may say that there is plenty of literature available on "thought-transference" and allied subjects.[20] "But how can we picture such a mind?" exclaims the enquirer. Definitely we cannot think of it as having any material form, size, color, feel, taste, or smell. The fact is that "thinking" is of the life and "thought of" is of the matter. So the life or the mind proper is formless and is not an object of thought.

Now I have a compromise to suggest, which I think all will agree conforms to the reality of our general experience. When the camera takes the photograph all by itself in the dark, the matter in the form of the camera still retains the imprint of the

[20]See, however, especially Prof. Geley's *Clairvoyance and Materialization,* and the works of Dr. J. B. Rhine, of Duke University.

life which has acted upon it and given it that form. So the effect of the life is still there in the nature of what we may call a "material memory." Briefly, although the camera was formed or took form, or acquired its form under the influence or action of the life, in the shape of a thought, it still retains that form even though the thinking is now withdrawn. I believe that this method of nature has been classified by philosophers, as "objective idealism," because after the form has been produced by an action based upon an idea it retains its objectivity in the world even when the idea has ceased its operation. Reverse this, and you have "the world of the mind."

Now, that is important—just as there is objective ideating, so there is also an imprint upon our minds which leaves the form in the mind as "memory" even after the contact with that form is a thing of the past. Therefore, just as the effect of the ideas on the forms remains in the objective field, so the effect of the forms on the mind remains in the subjective field. Therefore, with the eyes shut one can think about the objects of the world which one has seen. This can be called "the screen of the mind"— screen in the sense of a screen in a cinema.

Let us go so far as to say that the expression of an idea in form will have faithfulness to the idea only in the degree to which the action has been perfect, so also the representation of an object in the mind will be accurate, clear and strong only as a result of accurate, clear and strong perception, observation, concentration or whatever we may call the quality of attention that the mind has given to it.

My next point is that this association or interaction of world and mind provides a mutual and lasting benefit to each. I will venture to say that the world is richer and finer on account of the works of man. A garden *is* better than a jungle. A house *is* better than a cave. A picture *is* better than an accidental splodge of mud on a rock. I say this in terms of evolution: there *has* been some increase of both heterogeneity and cohesion in the world of material forms because of the operation of mind upon that matter and those forms. I do not say this is so in the grand mass, but in the spots where mankind dwells.

The converse also is true: there *has* been some improvement in the ideas in the mind and in that mind itself because of its perception of the objective forms in the world. How so? This psychological process is very familiar to all of us. The mind is not at first so clever that it can make and hold steady a thought of its own. There is some vagueness, some wavering, some vacillation about it. But if that mind proceeds to action, and tries to represent its thought in a form there is at once a steadying effect. The form stands there and the mind can look at it—closely, long and steadily if it so wishes. It can thus see the excellencies and the imperfections of it, and it can then proceed to improve upon it.

In this manner ideas in the mind are clarified by reference to facts. It is not merely that knowledge in the mind is *increased* by the careful observation of facts, but that in this very process the instrument of knowledge—the mind—is improved. It is seen to grow by use or exercise, and all the better so when it is provided with the large quantity of orderly material which nature presents so profusely for our inspection. Thus mind grows as muscle grows, but it seems to have less limitation or a more prodigious capacity. Think of Alekhine, who was able to play about thirty games of chess all at once without seeing any of the boards, do this with experts and win nearly all the games!

Further, it is not only in the matter of dealing with a variety and quantity of facts that the mind increases in power. Still more valuable to us is the increase in quality, by which I mean the very status of our consciousness and awareness. The only way in which I have felt able to express this difference in *quality* up to now is by comparing the power or intensity of it with different kinds of light, such as that from a taper, a candle, an oil lamp, a gas flame, an incandescent mantle, an electric bulb and an arc light. This in the mind is a state of being more alive, just as radiant health in the body is a state of being more alive than is common dullness of condition due to untrained or unintelligent eating, working, resting and breathing.

Although we are now concerned with the fact that the outside world helps us to steady, clarify and classify our thoughts, we may well pause to observe also that these varied surroundings provide an incentive to the mind's activity as well as to its clarity and volume. Yet in this we cannot reckon without the impulse which is in the mind itself. The mind is interested in things. Why? Because they provide an increase in our very sense of being; they enable us to be more than we were the moment before. It is this enjoyment of more being which is behind the mind, supporting and promoting mental interests.

I will not labor the point here, but I will point out that our life consists of being, doing and having, and yet the doings and havings are only interesting because they minister to our sense of being. We do not want to own cars, houses, and money in the bank; we want to *be* the owners of cars, houses and money in the bank. We do not want to do gardening, reading or mathematics; we want to *be* the doers of these acts. We want the enhancement of our consciousness or sense of being. I have already mentioned the little boy who did not like ice-cream, nor even the taste of it, but liked the consciousness of the taste of the ice-cream. The ego—in a good sense—is there, behind all these activities. He is the consciousness in the life, and is no doubt the source of the coherence referred to in our definition of evolution—a coherence which we cannot account for by any description or definition of matter.

We may now take a further step in our study of life and its environment. The things or forms which are so precious and valuable to us are only part of the world, not the whole of it. There are also other living beings all around us—an immense profusion and variety of them. Let us first consider the things which these other beings have brought into the world. For the most part the sub-human life around us has not been creative in the department of producing new objects. That has been the province of man, because of his more developed mind. If we came to an island and found a lot of clocks and watches lying about, and decrepit boats and deserted huts, we would say, "Men have been here," but we could only judge that animals had been there by remnants of their bodies, bleached bones, fossils and perhaps a beaver's dam, a few broken bird's nests and worm casts. Our association with animals is much more with the animals themselves than with their works. It is otherwise in the case of our association with other men; it is much more with their works than with them. Even when we meet one, we see very much more clothing than man. And we are always estimating people by what they have surrounded and enveloped themselves with. This is well, is it not, for we are thus much more acquainted with their minds (through their doings) than with their bodies. And so we obtain much more education from them than if it were otherwise.

In the case of the animals and the plants we are much more acquainted with their bodies than with their minds. Also, it seems, the simplicity of their minds, as compared with ours, offers us very little material for our education. But their bodies are so varied—due to their adaptation to circumstances for the enjoyment of living in a great variety of ways—that they present us with a panorama of immense interest and enrichment to the mind.

Now it must be said that our association with plants and animals and men (them and their works) is far more pleasurable, because more enriching, than our association with mere objects. One recalls the observation of Alexander Selkirk in this connection. He was monarch of all he surveyed, but alone, and found that he would rather live in the midst of alarms than "dwell in this horrible place."

This is emphatically and profoundly true, even though we do not see the life of other beings, but only their bodies, from which we infer their feelings and thoughts. This is not such a disadvantage as might seem at first sight, or rather first thought, because those bodies are their actions representing the well-formed, preserved and cherished contents or portions of their minds. Clothes may not make the man, but they can tell us what he is—a fop, a coward, a sluggard perhaps—better than he himself can do in his words or his thoughts, better in fact than he can tell himself what he is. So do we also know ourselves best through our bodies and our actions.

This rich and varied contact with other minds, although indirect, is incredibly valuable and rewarding, in the field of knowledge and in the field of action. It is the most precious thing in our lives. The benefits we derive from contact with mere objects cannot be compared with those we obtain from association with other minds. I mean material benefits, as well as mental. To this we must add pleasures, and shall I say happiness as well, since happiness arises not so much in the enjoyment of things as in the enjoyment of companionship. Need I elaborate this idea? The little child finds a funny spider, runs with it to mother, and says, "Look, mother!" The mother's interest and enjoyment gives the pleasure new quality.

Nothing is itself alone. This new quality due to companionship is not incidental. It *is* an enhancement of one's being. Readers of this may be reminded of Emerson's poem "Each and All."

This fact of unity in diversity, if properly meditated upon, and contemplated can, I am sure, give us a clue to the state of nirvana, in which separateness is eliminated—separateness and absences of all kinds, in both space and time, and nothing is lost or eliminated.

This is the reverse of negativeness. In such a state hearing, feeling, touching, tasting and smelling and whatever other senses there may be would be unseparated, and there would be no need for mind to perform its present unionising of what is now experienced separately in space and time. The nature of law is also a subject for meditation, as indicating this transcendency of separateness, for laws appear "out of nowhere" wherever they are apposite, without transference or loss by use, without creation or dissolution. They are not expendable as energy is. And so there remains one final truth awaiting us, that when "the dewdrop slips into the shining sea" we shall find that "the universe grows I" and only the illusions and frustrations of separateness have been dissolved.